Fundamentals **Success**

A Q & A Review Applying Critical Thinking to Test Taking

FOURTH EDITION

Fundamentals **Success**

A Q & A Review Applying Critical Thinking to Test Taking

FOURTH EDITION

Patricia M. Nugent, RN, MA, MS, EdD
Professor Emeritus
Adjunct Professor
Nassau Community College
Garden City, New York
Private Practice—President of Nugent Books, Inc.

Barbara A. Vitale, RN, MA
Professor Emeritus
Nassau Community College
Garden City, New York
Private Practice—Professional Resources for Nursing

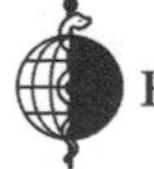

F.A. Davis Company • Philadelphia

F. A. Davis Company
1915 Arch Street
Philadelphia, PA 19103
www.fadavis.com

Printed in the United States of America

Last digit indicates print number: 10 9 8 7 6 5 4 3 2 1

Publisher, Nursing: Robert G. Martone
Director of Content Development: Darlene D. Pedersen
Content Project Manager: Jacalyn C. Clay
Electronic Project Editor: Sandra A. Glennie
Design and Illustration Manager: Carolyn O'Brien

ISBN: 978-0-8036-4414-4

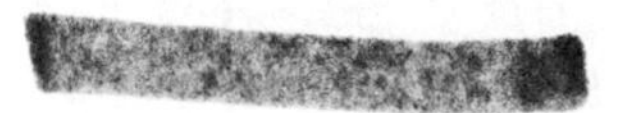

Dedicated to

Neil Nugent
and
Joseph Vitale

For their love, support, sense of humor, enthusiasm for life,
and attempts to keep our compulsive natures under control.

Reviewers

Cynthia Aaron
Stillman College
Tuscaloosa, Alabama

Carol Alexander
Palm Beach State College
Lake Worth, Florida

Bonnie Allen
Illinois Central College
East Peoria, Illinois

Cindy Baker
Murray State College
Tishoming, Oklahoma

Cynthia Bostick
California State University, Dominguez Hills
Carson, California

Barbara Bozicevich
Hibbing Community College
Hibbing, Minnesota

Barbara Britton
Fayetteville Technical Community College
Fayetteville, North Carolina

Christine Brooks
Palm Beach Atlantic University
West Palm Beach, Florida

Catherine Caston
Concordia University
Irvine, California

Amy C. Chavarria
South Texas College
McAllen, Texas

Rita Ciccone
Ohio Valley General Hospital
McKees Rocks, Pennsylvania

Cathy Coram
Pueblo Community College—Freemond Campus
Canon, City, Colorado

Kelli Davis
Gadsden State Community College
Centre, Alabama

Amanda Day
Academy of Medical and Health Science
Pueblo, Colorado

Donna Dexter
Citizens School of Nursing
New Kensington, Pennsylvania

Lori Evans
Greater Lowell Tech
Tyngsboro, Massachusetts

Vesta Fairley
Bishop State Community College
Mobile, Alabama

Cris Finn
Regis University
Denver, Colorado

Karen L. Fuqua
South Texas College
McAllen, Texas

Dawana Gibbs
College of Coastal Georgia
Brunswick, Georgia

Sharlene Georgesen
Morningside College
Sioux City, Iowa

Geraldine Valencia-Go
College of New Rochelle
New Rochelle, New York

Lois Gotes
Carl Albert State College
Poteau, Oklahoma

Deborah Henderson
Bay Path PN Program
Charlton, Massachusetts

Kara Hoffman
Ohio Valley General Hospital
McKees Rocks, Pennsylvania

Monica Holland
Oklahoma City Community College
Oklahoma City, Oklahoma

Anita Jones
Murray State College
Tishomingo, Oklahoma

Susan Karcher
Harold B. and Dorothy A. Snyder Schools
Plainfield, New Jersey

Kathleen Kavanagh
Felician College
Lodi, New Jersey

Elizabeth Kawecki
South University West Palm Beach
Royal Palm Beach, Florida

Patricia Kelly
Saint Xavier University
Chicago, Illinois

Maggie King
Xavier University
Cincinnati, Ohio

Mary Kovarna
Morningside College
Sioux City, Iowa

Christine Kowal
Cumberland University
Lebanon, Tennessee

Rhonda Lansdell
Northeast Mississippi Community College
Booneville, Mississippi

Tracy Lopez
Dona Ana Community College
Las Cruces, New Mexico

Judy Maynard
Fayetteville Technical Community College
Fayetteville, North Carolina

Tammie McCoy
Mississippi University for Women
Columbus, Mississippi

Victoria Newton
Northeastern Hospital School of Nursing
Philadelphia, Pennsylvania

Amanda M. Reynolds
Grambling State University
Grambling, Louisiana

Deborah A. Roberts
Sonoma State
Rohnert Park, California

Jane Rosati
Daytona State College
Daytona Beach, Florida

Jeffrey Ross
Bainbridge College
Bainbridge, Georgia

Laura Saucer
South University Montgomery
Montgomery, Alabama

Beverly Schaefer
Ursuline College
Pepper Pike, Ohio

Dianne Scott
Northwest Mississippi Community College
Senatobia, Mississippi

Patty Shanaberger
El Paso Community College
El Paso, Texas

Patricia A. Sharpnack
Ursuline College
Pepper Pike, Ohio

Jeanne Siegel
University of Miami
Miami, Florida

Nancy Simpson
University of New England
Portland, Maine

Julia Skrabal
BryanLGH College of Health Sciences
Lincoln, Nebraska

Pamela Sonney
Durham Technical Community College
Durham, North Carolina

Susan Stone
Valencia Community College
Orlando, Florida

Mary Tan
Holmes Community College
Ridgeland, Mississippi

Lois Thomas
Roxborough Memorial Hospital School of Nursing
Philadelphia, Pennsylvania

Diane Thorup
Cumberland University
Lebanon, Tennessee

Lynne Tier
Florida Hospital College of Health Sciences
Orlando, Florida

Carol Tingle
Baton Rouge General MC School of Nursing
Baton Rouge, Louisiana

Dianna Tison
University of the Incarnate Word
San Antonio, Texas

June Vermillion
New Mexico State University
Las Cruces, New Mexico

Robin Weaver
Ohio Valley Hospital School of Nursing
McKees Rocks, Pennsylvania

Kathleen Weigel
North Dakota State College of Science
Wahpeton, North Dakota

Lisa White
Arnot Ogden School of Nursing
Elmira, New York

Jo-Ann Whitesell
St. John's River Community College
Palatka, Florida

Patricia Wolpert
Mulhenberg Snyder School of Nursing
Plainfield, New Jersey

Jean Zlomke
Laramie County Community College
Cheyenne, Wyoming

Item Writers

Mary Ann Hellmer Saul, PhD, RN, CNE
Professor
Nassau Community College
Garden City, New York

Michael W. Mangino, Jr., RN, NP-Psychiatry
Associate Professor
Suffolk Community College
Selden, New York

Medical Consultant

Joanne M. Vitale, RPA-C
Physician Assistant
Romanelli Cosmetic Surgery
Huntington, New York
Huntington Hospital
North Shore LIJ Health System

Acknowledgments

Many people at F. A. Davis were essential to the production of this book. We especially want to thank Bob Martone, Publisher for Nursing, whose skills of listening and focusing as well as expertise in publishing were instrumental to the production of this edition. He has shared our passion for this project through seven editions and we value his knowledge and especially his friendship over the last 23 years. We thank the entire F.A. Davis staff who competently transformed our manuscript into a book. We salute Jacalyn Clay, Project Editor, for her editorial expertise. She always was available, answered our every request, and supported and encouraged us throughout the revision. We also thank Lisa Thompson, Production Editor, who managed every detail skillfully and was never ruffled; Julia Curcio, Content Project Manager who expertly managed all the illustrations with finesse; and Holly Lukens, copy editor, who was phenomenal with the details of grammar and content. A special thanks to F. A. Davis sales representatives who have done a spectacular job of highlighting the strengths of our texts to nursing faculty.

Special recognition goes to all the nursing students and faculty who participated in field-testing sessions and focus groups for their commitment to excellence and generosity in sharing their time, energy, and intellect. We also thank the nursing educators who reviewed manuscript that provided feedback for us to fine tune the content and its presentation. Finally, and most importantly, we thank our husbands, Neil and Joseph, for their love and support, which were essential to the revision of this book. They are loved and appreciated by us.

A Message to Nursing Educators

Nurses are required to use critical thinking in every domain of nursing practice.

- Accrediting bodies of educational programs have increased the emphasis on maximizing the cognitive abilities of learners.
- Licensing examinations are designed to evaluate the test taker's ability to engage in clinical reasoning.
- Agency accrediting bodies have developed standards that require creative, evidenced-based practice.
- Health care, health-care environments, and technology have increased in complexity, requiring sophisticated health-care practitioners.

The premise of this book is based on the beliefs that:

- People use critical thinking all the time in their daily lives.
- People can enhance their critical-thinking skills.
- Students can use critical-thinking skills when taking a nursing examination.
- Nurses continue to use critical thinking in their professional lives.

How can nursing educators help students think critically?

- Help students develop their critical-thinking abilities through the information contained in Chapter 1.
  - Help students identify and develop their cognitive and personal competencies by exploring the Helix of Critical Thinking.
  - Support students who are maximizing their critical-thinking abilities by being positive, reflective, inquisitive, and creative.
  - Help students use the RACE Model, a formula for applying critical thinking, when answering nursing questions.
- Encourage students to practice test taking by answering the questions and reviewing the answers and their rationales in Chapters 2 through 5 to:
  - Reinforce what they know.
  - Learn new information.
  - Identify what still needs to be learned.
  - Set priorities for future learning.
- Have students practice answering alternate format questions (e.g., exhibit, multiple response, drag-and-drop [ordered response], hot spot, fill-in-the-blank, audio, and items using a chart, table, or graphic image) presented in Chapter 6 to develop critical-thinking skills in relation to questions that authentically evaluate unique nursing interventions (e.g., calculations, setting priorities, interpreting sounds, and analyzing data from multiple sources).
- Have students practice taking comprehensive examinations with integrated fundamental content gleaned from sub-units of nursing information. Chapter 7, Comprehensive Final Book Exam, has a 100-item integrated examination. The RACE Model is applied to every question on this 100-item examination. This role-models the clinical reasoning that can be employed when answering a nursing test question.
- Encourage students to practice answering nursing questions on the computer. In addition to this book's 100-item Comprehensive Final Book Exam, DavisPlus.com has two accompanying 75-item integrated tests. The student can access these tests or they can self-select questions based on content area.

- Encourage students to review the keywords at the beginning of each clinical sub-unit in Chapters 2 through 5. Knowing the definition of these words and understanding concepts and principles associated with them will build a theoretical base for answering the questions in the content area.
- Encourage students, particularly those who speak English as a second language, to learn the words in the Glossary of English Words Commonly Encountered on Nursing Examinations. This will allow students taking a test to concentrate on nursing content rather than being distracted by a lack of comprehension of English words.

A Message to Nursing Students

If you are similar to the average nursing student, you read assigned chapters in your textbook and articles in nursing journals, review your classroom notes, complete computer instruction programs related to nursing content, practice nursing skills in a simulated laboratory, and apply in the clinical area what you have learned. All these activities are excellent ways for you to expand and strengthen your theoretical base and become a safe practitioner of nursing. However, these activities may not be enough for you to be successful when taking a nursing examination. You need to practice test taking as early as possible in your program of study with questions appropriate for your level of nursing education. In addition, you must be aware of, strengthen, and expand your cognitive competencies (intellectual reasoning skills) and personal competencies (individual attitudes or qualities) reflected in **The Helix of Critical Thinking** and then utilize these components of critical thinking when answering nursing questions.

Nursing students keep making the same statements:

- I need more examples of nursing test questions, especially alternate format items.
- I need to practice taking nursing examinations on the computer.
- I need to learn how to answer a nursing test question.
- **I need to pass my nursing examinations!**

This book addresses these needs.

WHY YOU SHOULD READ THIS TEXTBOOK

FEATURES	BENEFITS
A discussion of maximizing your critical-thinking abilities, including the attitudes and qualities of successful critical thinkers and strategies to overcome barriers to critical thinking.	This discussion provides a basis for a self-assessment in relation to these qualities and introduces strategies that you can use to overcome barriers to your critical thinking. This discussion should motivate you to maintain a positive mental attitude and be reflective, inquisitive, and creative when thinking.
Keyword list at the beginning of each chapter that includes vocabulary, and nursing/medical terminology, essential to the content of nursing.	These words encourage you to focus on the critical components of a topic of study. Understanding these critical words expands your theoretical base and provides a strong foundation for more advanced concepts.
The **RACE Model** is introduced and applied to a variety of sample questions and every question in the 100-item Comprehensive Final Book Exam.	These specific examples model the critical-thinking processes involved when answering increasingly complex questions in nursing. This facilitates imitating the critical-thinking activities used in answering questions in the practice of nursing. Ultimately, when you can critically analyze a question and answer it correctly, you will feel empowered, and your test anxiety will decrease.

continued

continued

Over 1,300 quality fundamentals of nursing questions.	These questions allow you to practice test taking and apply critical thinking via the RACE Model. This practice should increase your critical-thinking skills, promote your self-confidence, build your stamina when taking tests, and reduce test anxiety.
Over 475 questions with formats other than multiple choice. More than 35—Chart exhibit items 22—Hot-spot items 35—Illustration/graphic items 58—Drag and drop items 43—Fill-in-the-blank items 286—Multiple-response items 35.5% of questions in the text are alternate item formats.	These questions will: Expose you to the alternate types of question formats that appear in NCLEX examinations, particularly the new audio question. Allow you to practice nursing questions that incorporate multiple-response, fill-in-the-blank, hot-spot, chart/exhibit, drop and drag (ordered response), and audio items and questions that refer to an image such as an illustration, chart, table, or photograph. Reduce anxiety concerning alternate formats you will be confronted with on the NCLEX examination.
Rationales for the correct and incorrect answers for every question.	Reviewing the rationales for every question will: Reinforce what you know—this increases trust in your ability and promotes a sense of security. Teach you new information—this increases your knowledge and builds self-confidence. Identify what you still need to learn—this focuses and prioritizes your study activities so that the return on your effort is maximized.
100-item Comprehensive Final Book Exam	This provides you with an opportunity to integrate fundamental content learned in sub-units of study into one examination. The RACE Model is applied to every question to demonstrate the critical thinking that is employed when answering nursing test questions.
Two 75-item Comprehensive Exit Exams available on DavisPlus.com.	These provide you with an opportunity to practice test taking on a computer. They allow you to take two comprehensive examinations that integrate sub-units of fundamentals of nursing content.
Create your own test accessing the questions available from this text on DavisPlus.com based on self-selected areas within Integrated Processes, Client Need, Cognitive Level, and/or Difficulty Level.	This allows you to focus on questions in a unit of study, steps in the nursing process, client need category, or cognitive domain of your choice. This allows you then to design a test with a lower level of difficulty and then to move onto questions that are on a higher level of difficulty. This supports confidence.
Glossary that identifies and defines ordinary English words that appear frequently in nursing examinations.	Familiarity with these words reduces the challenge of a test question because you can center your attention on the theoretical content presented in the question.

To increase your knowledge of fundamentals of nursing theory and be successful on nursing examinations, it is important for you to use this book—***Fundamentals Success: A Q & A Review Applying Critical Thinking to Test Taking, Fourth Edition.*** Although this book is valuable for all nursing students regardless of their level of nursing education, it is essential for beginning nursing students. The related knowledge, attitudes, and skills that you develop early in your fundamental nursing courses influence your present and future educational performance. A house will stand and survive only when it is built on a strong foundation. The same concept can be applied to your nursing education. The components of a strong foundation in nursing are a comprehensive understanding of the fundamentals of nursing theory, well-developed critical-thinking abilities, and an inventory of strategies for successful test taking.

Another textbook you may find helpful toward maximizing your success when preparing for and taking examinations in nursing is ***Test Success: Test-Taking Techniques for Beginning Nursing Students*** (Nugent & Vitale, F. A. Davis Company). This book focuses on empowerment, critical thinking, study techniques, the multiple-choice question, the nursing process, test-taking techniques, testing formats other than multiple-choice questions (including alternate formats on NCLEX examinations), and computer applications in education and evaluation. It also contains hundreds of fundamentals of nursing questions, of which more than 25% are alternate format items. Every question has test-taking techniques and rationales for correct and incorrect answers. It includes a 100-item Comprehensive Final Book Exam and a two 75-item Comprehensive Exit Exams available on DavisPlus.com.

We are firm believers in the old sayings, "You get out of it what you put into it!" and "Practice makes perfect!" The extent of your learning, the attitudes you develop, and the skills you acquire depend on the energy you are willing to expend. It is our belief that if you give this book your best effort, you will strengthen and expand your theoretical foundation of fundamentals of nursing and your critical-thinking abilities in testing situations. We expect your efforts to be rewarded with success on your nursing examinations!

Figure Credits

Chapter 1

Page 20 from Vitale [2013]. NCLEX-RN Notes, 2nd ed. Philadelphia: F.A. Davis Company, with permission.

Chapter 2

Page 33, 42 from Dunn, H. L. High level wellness for man and society. American Journal of Public Health. 1959; 49(6): 786–788, with permission.

Chapter 3

Page 133, 140, 163 from Wilkinson and Treas [2011]. Fundamentals of Nursing, 2nd ed. Vol. 1. Philadelphia, F.A. Davis Company, with permission.

Chapter 4

Page 197, (top) from Dillon [2007]. Nursing Health Assessment, 2nd ed. Philadelphia: F.A. Davis Company, with permission.

Page 197 (bottom), 206 Courtesy of Kingfisher Regional Hospital. Kingfisher, OK.

Page 212 From Wilkinson and Van Leuven [2007]. Fundamentals of Nursing. Philadelphia: F.A. Davis Company, with permission.

Page 211, 219, 227, 229, 234, 237, 248, 254: From Wilkinson and Treas [2011]. Fundamentals of Nursing, 2nd ed. Vol. 1. Philadelphia, F.A. Davis Company, with permission.

Page 243, 246, 257 from Nugent and Vitale [2014]. Fundamentals of Nursing: Content Review Plus Practice Questions. Philadelphia: F.A. Davis Company, with permission.

Chapter 5

Page 321, 330, 425, 436 from Nugent and Vitale [2014]. Fundamentals of Nursing: Content Review Plus Practice Questions. Philadelphia: F.A. Davis Company, with permission.

Page 323, 341 from Burton and Ludwig [2011]. Fundamentals of Nursing Care. Philadelphia: F.A. Davis Company, with permission.

Page 340, 373, 424 from Wilkinson and Treas [2011]. Fundamentals of Nursing, 2nd ed. Vol. 2. Philadelphia, F.A. Davis Company, with permission.

Page 390, 398 from Phillips [2010]. Manual of I.V. Therapeutics: Evidence-Based Practice for Infusion Therapy, 5th ed. Philadelphia: F.A. Davis Company, with permission.

Page 405 FLACC Behavioral Scale. © 2002 The Regents of the University of Michigan. All Rights Reserved.

Page 423 from Aldrete, J. A. [1995]. Reprinted from Journal of Clinical Anesthesia, Vol. 7/ Issue 1, Post-anesthesia recovery score revisited, pp.89–91, with permission from Elsevier.

Chapter 6

Page 440 (bottom), 441 (bottom), 442 (top), 460 (top left and right), 461 (top left) from Burton and Ludwig [2011]. Fundamentals of Nursing Care. Philadelphia: F.A. Davis Company, with permission.

Page 443 (bottom), 449, 461 (bottom right) from Wilkinson and Treas [2011]. Fundamentals of Nursing, 2nd ed. Vol. 2. Philadelphia, F.A. Davis Company, with permission.

Chapter 7

Page 478 from Wilkinson and Treas [2011]. Fundamentals of Nursing, 2nd ed. Vol. 2. Philadelphia, F.A. Davis Company, with permission.

Page 480, 483, 510, 519 from Burton and Ludwig [2011]. Fundamentals of Nursing Care. Philadelphia: F.A. Davis Company, with permission.

Contents

1 Fundamentals of Critical Thinking Related to Test Taking

INTRODUCTION

To prepare for writing this chapter we did what all writers should do. We performed a detailed search of the literature about critical thinking, we reviewed all the significant materials that related to test taking or nursing practice, and we wrote an outline for a comprehensive discussion of critical thinking in relation to nursing examinations. The introductory section of the chapter was to be titled "The Historical Perspective of Critical Thinking." When we typed the chapter heading and reread it, we had written "Hysterical" instead of "Historical." Having a relatively good sense of humor and the ability to laugh at ourselves, our response was peals of laughter. We realized that this was a Freudian slip! Loosely defined, a *Freudian slip* occurs when unconscious mental processes result in a verbal statement that reflects more accurately the true feelings of the speaker than does the originally intended statement. Being true believers in the statement that *all behavior has meaning*, we could not continue until we explored why we wrote what we wrote.

When we looked up the word *hysterical* in the dictionary, its definitions were *an uncontrollable outburst of emotion* or *out of control* and *extremely comical* or *hilarious*. Associating the word "hysterical" with the concept of critical thinking raised two thoughts. Are we overwhelmed, frantic, and out of control when considering the relationship between critical thinking and nursing, or do we find this relationship funny, comical, and hilarious? If you feel overwhelmed, frenzied, or out of control when considering critical thinking, carefully read the section in this chapter titled *Be Positive: You Can Do It!* When we personalized the word to our own experiences, we recalled that when we believe that something is funny, our internal communication is "Isn't that hysterically funny?" So, now we were faced with the task of exploring why we thought reviewing the historical perspective of critical thinking was so funny or why it could be overwhelming. We actually spent several hours pursuing this goal. At the completion of this process, we arrived at three conclusions:

- The words "critical thinking" are just buzzwords. *Critical thinking* is a skill that we all possess uniquely, and we use this skill routinely in all the activities of our daily living. It is funny to profess that critical thinking is something new and different.
- Who cares about the historical perspectives of critical thinking! Information about the abstract topic of critical thinking must be presented in a manner that the information learned today can be implemented tomorrow.
- Feelings of being overwhelmed can be conquered because critical-thinking abilities can be enhanced.

Definition of Critical Thinking

As we sat back and reflected on our morning's work in relation to Alfaro-LeFevre's (1995) definition of critical thinking, we recognized and appreciated the fact that we had been thoroughly involved with critical thinking. We had:

- Engaged in purposeful, goal-directed thinking.
- Aimed to make judgments based on evidence (fact) rather than conjecture (guesswork).
- Employed a process based on principles of science (e.g., problem solving, decision making).

- Used strategies (e.g., metacognition, reflection, Socratic questioning) that maximized our human potential and compensated for problems caused by human nature.

Critical thinking is a cognitive strategy by which you reflect on and analyze your thoughts, actions, and decisions. Critical thinking often is integrated into traditional linear processes. Linear processes usually follow a straight line, with a beginning and a product at the end. Some linear-like processes, such as the nursing process, are considered cyclical because they repeat themselves. Some formal reasoning processes include the following:

- **Problem Solving** involves identifying a problem, exploring alternative interventions, implementing selected interventions, and arriving at the end product, which is a solution to the problem.
- **Decision Making** involves carefully reviewing significant information, using methodical reasoning, and arriving at the end product, which is a decision.
- **Diagnostic Reasoning** involves collecting information, correlating the collected information to standards, identifying the significance of the collected information, and arriving at the end product, which is a conclusion or nursing diagnosis.
- **The Scientific Method** involves identifying a problem to be investigated, collecting data, formulating a hypothesis, testing the hypothesis through experimentation, evaluating the hypothesis, and arriving at the end product, which is acceptance or rejection of the hypothesis.
- **The Nursing Process** involves collecting information (Assessment); determining significance of information and making a nursing diagnosis (Analysis/Diagnosis); identifying priorities, goals, expected outcomes, and nursing interventions (Planning); carrying out nursing interventions (Implementation/Intervention); and assessing the patient's response to interventions and comparing the actual outcomes with expected outcomes (Evaluation), ultimately to arrive at the end product of meeting a person's needs.

Each of these methods of manipulating and processing information incorporates critical thinking. They all are influenced by intellectual standards, such as being focused, methodical, deliberate, logical, relevant, accurate, precise, clear, comprehensive, creative, and reflective. It is helpful to incorporate critical thinking into whatever framework or structure that works for you.

The purpose of this discussion is to impress on you that you:

- Use critical thinking in your personal life.
- Will continue to use critical thinking in your professional life.
- Should enhance your critical-thinking abilities when studying.
- Can employ critical-thinking skills when taking a nursing examination.

In an attempt to make the abstract aspects of critical thinking more concrete, we have schematically represented our concept of critical thinking by the **Helix of Critical Thinking.** In Figure 1–1, the Helix of Critical Thinking has been unwound and enlarged so that the components of the cognitive competencies and personal competencies can be viewed easily. The cognitive competencies are the intellectual or reasoning processes employed when thinking. The personal competencies are the characteristics or attitudes of the individual thinker. These lists of competencies represent the cognitive abilities or personal qualities commonly associated with critical thinkers. No one possesses all of these competencies, and you may identify competencies that you possess that are not on these lists. The lists are not all inclusive. Make lists of your own cognitive and personal competencies. Your lists represent your repertoire or inventory of thinking skills. As you gain knowledge and experience, your lists will expand. The more cognitive and personal competencies you possess, the greater your potential to think critically.

The Helix of Critical Thinking, when wound (Fig. 1–2), demonstrates the integration of cognitive competencies and personal competencies essential to thinking critically. Not all of these competencies are used in every thinking situation. You can pick or choose from them as from a smorgasbord when you are confronted with situations that require critical thinking. Initially, you may have to stop and consciously consider what cognitive competencies (i.e., intellectual skills) or personal competencies (i.e., abilities, attitudes) to use. As you gain knowledge and experience and move toward becoming an expert critical thinker, the use of these competencies will become second nature. The Helix will contract or expand depending on the competencies you use in a particular circumstance. In addition, there is constant interaction among cognitive competencies, among personal competencies, and between cognitive competencies and personal competencies.

The interactive nature of the Helix of Critical Thinking and the Nursing Process is demonstrated in Figure 1–3. **The Nursing Process is a critical thinking framework that involves assessing and analyzing human responses to plan and implement nursing care that meets patient needs as evidenced by the evaluation of patient outcomes.** The Nursing Process provides a precise framework in which purposeful thinking occurs.

Cognitive Competencies	Personal Competencies
Dissect	Thinking independently
Modify	Tolerant of ambiguity
Analyze	Self-confident
Interpret	Open-minded
Examine	Accountable
Correlate	Courageous
Synthesize	Persevering
Investigate	Imaginative
Recall facts	Disciplined
Categorize	Risk taking
Summarize	Committed
Understand	Inquisitive
Demonstrate	Motivated
Self-examine	Confident
Translate data	Reflective
Query evidence	Objective
Make inferences	Authentic
Manipulate facts	Assertive
Present arguments	Intuitive
Establish priorities	Rational
Make generalizations	Creative
Compare and contrast	Humble
Determine significance	Curious
Determine implications	Honest
Determine consequences	Moral

Figure 1–1. The Helix of Critical Thinking is schematically elongated to demonstrate the components of cognitive competencies and personal competencies. The more cognitive competencies and personal competencies a person possesses, the greater the potential the person has to think critically.

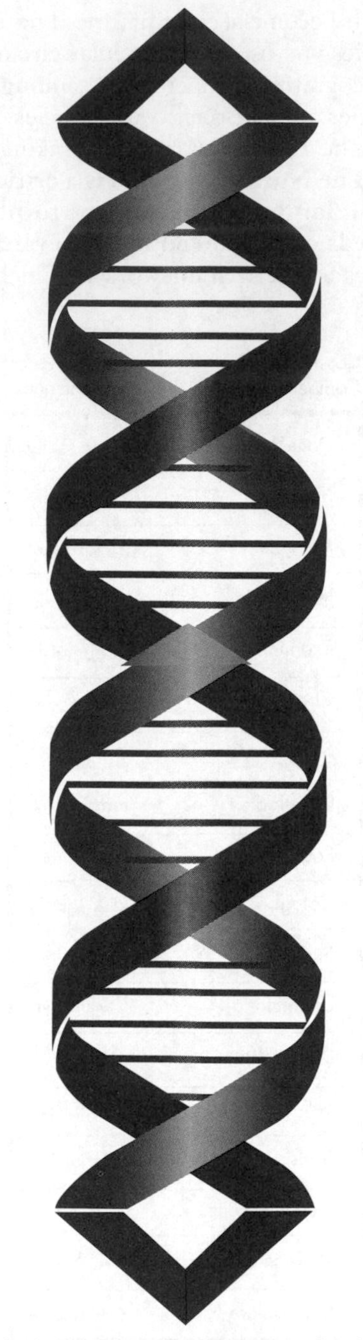

Figure 1–2. The Helix of Critical Thinking demonstrates the interwoven relationship between cognitive competencies and personal competencies essential to thinking critically. Throughout the thinking process there is constant interaction among cognitive competencies, among personal competencies, and between cognitive and personal competencies.

Critical thinking is an essential component within, between, and among the phases of the Nursing Process. Different combinations of cognitive and personal competencies may be used during different phases of the Nursing Process.

The interactive nature of the Helix of Critical Thinking and the Problem-Solving Process is demonstrated in Figure 1–4. **The Problem-Solving Process is a dynamic, linear process that has a beginning and an end, with a resolution of the identified problem.** It provides a progressive step-by-step method in which goal-directed thinking occurs. Critical thinking is an essential component within and between the steps of the Problem-Solving Process, and different combinations of cognitive and personal competencies may be used during the various steps involved.

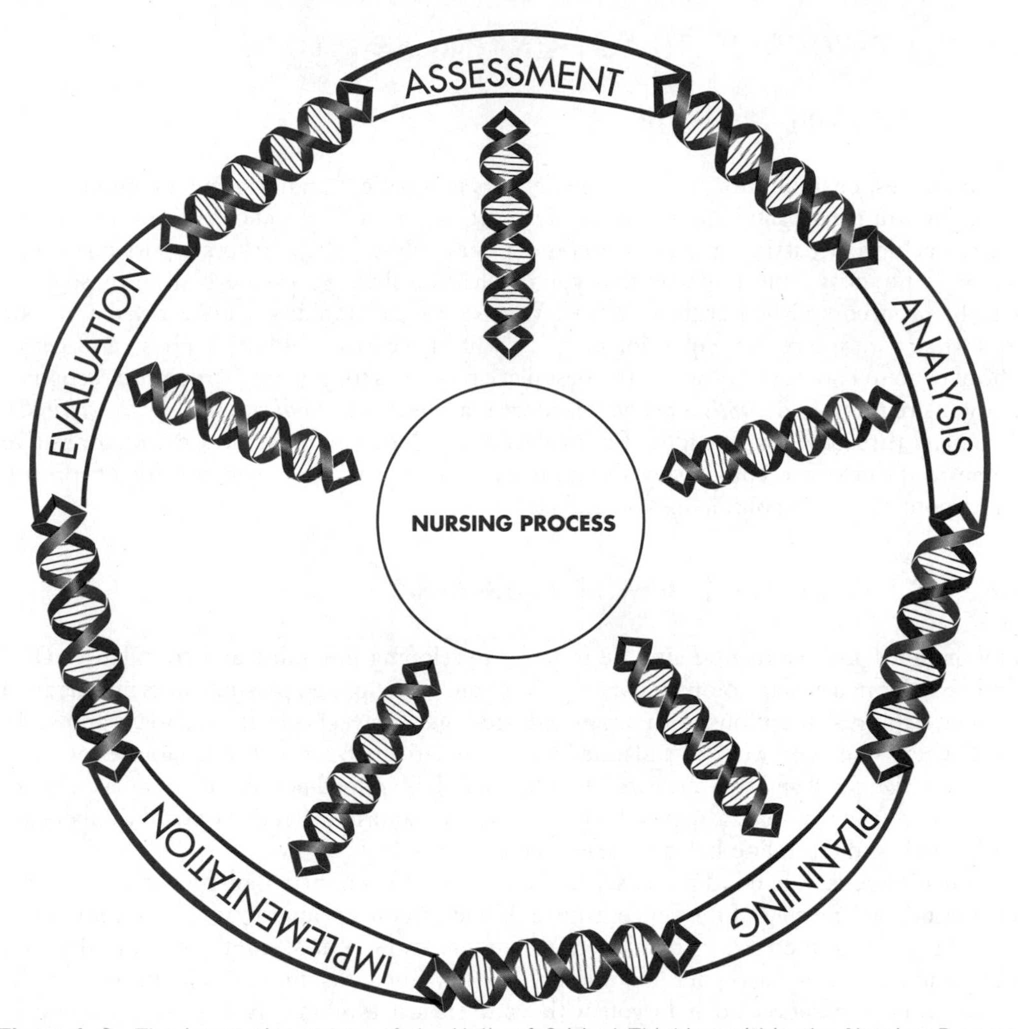

Figure 1–3. The interactive nature of the Helix of Critical Thinking within the Nursing Process. The Nursing Process is a dynamic, cyclical process in which each phase interacts with and is influenced by the other phases of the process. Critical thinking is an essential component within, between, and among phases of the Nursing Process. Different combinations of cognitive and personal competencies may be used during the different phases of the Nursing Process.

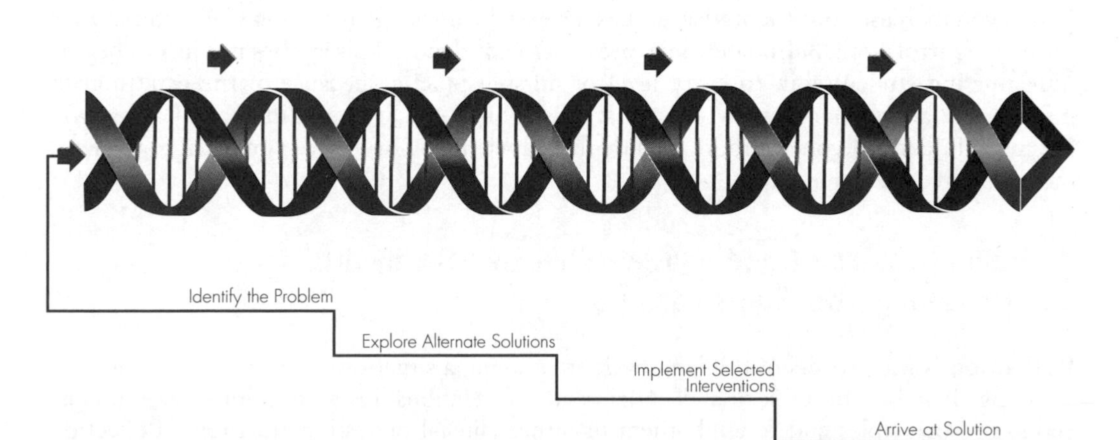

Figure 1–4. The interactive nature of the Helix of Critical Thinking within the Problem-Solving Process. The Problem-Solving Process is a dynamic, linear process that has a beginning and an end, with the resolution of the identified problem. Different combinations of cognitive and personal competencies may be used during the different steps of the Problem-Solving Process.

MAXIMIZE YOUR CRITICAL-THINKING ABILITIES

Be Positive: You Can Do It!

Assuming responsibility for the care one delivers to a patient and desiring a commendable grade on a nursing examination raise anxiety because a lot is at stake: to keep the patient safe; to achieve a passing grade; to become a nurse ultimately; and to support one's self-esteem. The most important skill that you can learn to help you achieve all of these goals is to be an accomplished critical thinker. We use critical-thinking skills every day in our lives when we explore these questions: "What will I have for breakfast?" "How can I get to school from my home?" "Where is the best place to get gas for my car?" Once you recognize that you are *thinking critically* already, it is more manageable to *think* about *thinking critically*. If you feel threatened by the idea of critical thinking, then you must do something positive to confront the threat. You must be disciplined and work at increasing your sense of control, which contributes to confidence! *You can do it!*

OVERCOME BARRIERS TO A POSITIVE MENTAL ATTITUDE

Supporting a positive mental attitude requires developing discipline and confidence. **Discipline** is defined as self-command or self-direction. A disciplined person works in a planned manner, explores all options in an organized and logical way, checks for accuracy, and seeks excellence. When you work in a planned and systematic manner with conscious effort, you are more organized and therefore more disciplined. Disciplined people generally have more control over the variables associated with an intellectual task. Effective critical thinkers are disciplined, and discipline helps to develop confidence.

Confidence is defined as poise, self-reliance, or self-assurance. Confidence increases as one matures in the role of the student nurse. Understanding your strengths and limitations is the first step to increasing confidence. When you know your strengths you can draw on them, and when you know your limitations you know when it is time to seek out the instructor or another resource to help you with your critical thinking. Either way, you are in control! For example, ask the instructor for help when critically analyzing a case study, share with the instructor any concerns you have about a clinical assignment, and seek out the instructor in the clinical area when you feel the need for support. Failing to use your instructor is like putting your head in the sand. Learning needs must be addressed, not avoided. Although your instructor is responsible for your clinical practice and for stimulating your intellectual growth as a nursing student, you are the consumer of your nursing education. As the consumer, you must be an active participant in your own learning by ensuring that you get the assistance and experiences you need to build your abilities and confidence. When you increase your theoretical and experiential knowledge base, you will increase your sense of control, which ultimately increases your confidence. This applies not just to beginning nursing students but to every level of nursing practice because of the explosion in information and technology. When you are disciplined you are more in control, when you are more in control you are more confident, and when you are more confident you have a more positive mental attitude.

Be Reflective: You Need to Take One Step Backward Before Taking Two Steps Forward!

Reflection is the process of thinking back or recalling a situation or event to rediscover its meaning. It helps you to seek and understand the relationships among information, concepts, and principles and to apply them in future clinical or testing situations. Reflection can be conducted internally as quiet thoughtful consideration, in a one-on-one discussion with an instructor or another student, or in a group.

As a beginning nursing student, you are just starting to develop an experiential background from the perspective of a provider of nursing care. However, you have a wealth of experiences, personal and educational, that influence your development as a licensed nurse. Your personal experiences include activities using verbal and written communication, such as delegating tasks to family members or coworkers, setting priorities for daily activities, using mathematics when shopping or balancing a checkbook, and so on. A nursing program of study incorporates courses from a variety of other disciplines, such as anatomy and physiology, chemistry, physics, psychology, sociology, reading, writing, mathematics, and informatics. Every experience is a potential valuable resource for future learning. Recognize the value of the "you" you bring to your nursing education and incorporate it into your reflective processes.

Engaging in reflection is a highly individualized mental process. One form of reflection is writing a journal. A **journal** is an objective and subjective diary of your experiences. It is a chronicle that includes cognitive learning, feelings, and attitudes, and it requires you actively to develop skills related to assessing, exploring the meaning of critical incidents, documenting, developing insights into thoughts and actions that comprise clinical practice, and evaluating. Journal writing is a rich resource that provides a written record of where you have been, where you are, and where you are going. It helps you to incorporate experiences into the development of your professional being. After an examination, explore your feelings and attitudes regarding the experience. Be honest with yourself. Did you prepare adequately for the test? Did you find the content harder or easier than content on another test? Were you anxious before, during, or after the test and, if so, was your anxiety low, medium, or high? What would a low score or high score on the test mean to you? When you were confronted with a question that you perceived as difficult, how did you feel and how did you cope with the feeling? You do not necessarily have to ask yourself all of these questions. You should ask yourself those questions that have meaning for you.

Another form of reflection is making mental pictures. **Mental pictures** are visual images that can be recalled in the future. For example, when caring for a patient who has Parkinson's disease, compare the patient's signs and symptoms with the classic clinical manifestations associated with the disease. Then make a visual picture in your mind. Visualize the pill-rolling tremors, mask-like face, drooling, muscle rigidity, and so on, so that in the future you can recall the visual picture rather than having to remember a memorized list of symptoms.

Retrospective (after the event) reflection involves seeking an understanding of relationships between previously learned information and the application of this information in patient-care situations or testing experiences. This type of reflection helps you to judge your personal performance against standards of practice. A self-assessment requires the willingness to be open to identifying one's successful and unsuccessful interventions, strengths and weaknesses, and knowledge and lack of knowledge. The purpose of retrospective reflection is not to be judgmental or to second-guess decisions but rather to learn from the situation. The worth of the reflection depends on the abilities that result from it. When similar situations arise in subsequent clinical practice, previous actions that were reinforced or modified can be accessed to have a present successful outcome.

A *clinical postconference* is an example of retrospective reflection. Students often meet in a group (formally or informally) after a clinical experience to review the day's events. During the discussion, students have an opportunity to explore feelings and attitudes, consider interventions and alternative interventions, assess decision-making and problem-solving skills, identify how they and other students think through a situation, and so on. You can also review your own thinking when reviewing an experience with a patient by speaking aloud what you were thinking. For example:

> "When I went into the room to take my postoperative patient's vital signs I realized that the patient had an IV in the right arm. I knew that if I took a blood pressure in the arm with an IV it could interfere with the IV so I knew I had to take the blood pressure in the left arm. When I looked at my patient, he looked very pale and sweaty. I got a little nervous but I continued to get the other vital signs. I put the thermometer in the patient's mouth and started to take his pulse. It was very fast and I knew that this was abnormal so I paid special attention to its rhythm and volume. It was very thready but it was regular. The temperature and respirations were within the high side of the expected range."

A beginning nursing student may immediately respond by saying, "I don't know what is going on here so I better take this information to my instructor." A more advanced student could say, "What could be happening? Maybe the patient is bleeding or has an infection. I think I should inform my instructor but I'll inspect the incision first."

When you review an experience such as this example, you can identify your thinking skills. Taking the blood pressure in the left arm and assessing the rate, rhythm, and volume of the pulse were habits because you did not have to figure out a new method when responding to the situation. Remembering the expected range for the various vital signs used the thinking skill of total recall because you memorized and internalized these values. Determining further assessments after obtaining the vital signs required inquiry. You collected and analyzed information and did not take the vital sign results at face value. You recognized abnormalities and gaps in information, collected additional data, considered alternative conclusions, and identified alternative interventions.

Another example of retrospective reflection is reviewing an examination. When reviewing each question, determine why you got a question wrong. For example, several statements you could make are:

- I did not understand what the question was asking because of the English or medical vocabulary used in the question.
- I did not know or understand the content being tested.
- I knew the content being tested but I did not apply it correctly in the question.

When a limited English or medical vocabulary prevents you from answering a question correctly, you must spend time expanding this foundation. A list of English words that appear repeatedly in nursing examinations is included in a glossary at the end of this textbook. In addition, nursing/medical keyword lists have been included in each content area in this textbook. You can use these word lists to review key terminology used in nursing-related topics. To expand your vocabulary, keep English and medical dictionaries at your side when studying and look up new words, write flash cards for words you need to learn, and explore unfamiliar words with which you are confronted on tests.

When you answered a question incorrectly because you did not understand the content, make a list so that you can design a study session devoted to reviewing this information. This study session should begin with a brief review of what you do know about the topic (5 minutes or less). The majority of your efforts should be devoted to studying what you identified as what you need to know. You should do this after reviewing every test. This exercise is based on the axiom *strike while the iron is hot.* The test is over, so your anxiety level is reduced, and how nursing-related content is used in a test question is fresh in your mind. Study sessions that are goal directed tend to be more focused and productive.

When you know the content being tested but have applied the information incorrectly, it is an extremely frustrating experience. However, do not become discouraged. It is motivating to recognize that you actually know the content! Your next task is to explore how to tap into your knowledge successfully. Sometimes restating or summarizing what the question is asking places it into your own perspective, which helps to clarify the content in relation to the test question. Also, you can view the question in relation to specific past experiences or review the information in two different textbooks to obtain different perspectives on the same content. Another strategy to reinforce your learning is to use the left page of your notebook for taking class notes and leave the facing page blank. After an examination, use the blank page to make comments to yourself about how the content was addressed in test questions or add information from your textbook to clarify class notes. How to review thinking strategies in relation to cognitive levels of nursing questions is explored later in this chapter.

Examine your test-taking behaviors. For example, if you consistently changed your initial answers on a test, it is wise to explore what factors influenced you to change your answers. In addition, determine how many questions were converted to either right or wrong answers. The information you collect from this assessment should influence your future behaviors. If you consistently changed correct answers to incorrect answers, you should examine the factors that caused you to change your answers. If you changed incorrect answers to correct answers, you should identify what mental processes were used to arrive at your second choice so that you can use them the first time you look at a question.

Reflection is an essential component of all learning. How can you know where you are going without knowing where you have been? Therefore, to enhance your critical-thinking abilities you must *take one step backward before taking two steps forward!*

OVERCOME BARRIERS TO EFFECTIVE REFLECTION

Reflecting on your knowledge, strengths, and successes is easy, but reflecting on your lack of knowledge, weaknesses, and mistakes takes courage and humility. **Courage** is the attitude of confronting anything recognized as dangerous or difficult without avoiding or withdrawing from the situation. Courage is necessary because when people look at their shortcomings they tend to be judgmental and are their own worst critics. This type of negativity must be avoided because it promotes defensive thinking, interferes with the reception of new information, and limits self-confidence.

Humility is having a modest opinion of one's own abilities. Humility is necessary because it is important to admit your limitations. Only when you identify what you do and do not know can you make a plan to acquire the knowledge necessary to be successful on nursing examinations and practice safe nursing care. Arrogance or a "know-it-all" attitude can interfere with maximizing your potential. For example, when reviewing examinations with students, the students who benefit the most are the ones who are willing to listen to their peers or instructor as to why the correct answer is correct. The students who benefit the least are the ones who consistently and vehemently defend their wrong answers. A healthy amount of inquiry, thoughtful questioning, and not accepting statements at their face value are important critical-thinking competencies; however, self-righteous or obstructionist attitudes more often than not impede, rather than promote, learning.

Be Inquisitive: If You Don't Go There, You'll Never Get Anywhere!

To **inquire** means to question or investigate. The favorite words of inquisitive people are: *what, where, when,* and, most important, *how, why, if . . . then,* and *it depends.* When studying, ask yourself these words to delve further into a topic under consideration. The following are examples:

- You raise the head of the bed when a patient is short of breath. You recognize that this intervention will facilitate respirations. Ask yourself the question, "*How* does this intervention facilitate respirations?" The answer could be, "Raising the head of the bed allows the abdominal organs to drop by gravity, which reduces pressure against the diaphragm, which, in turn, permits maximal thoracic expansion."
- You insert an indwelling urinary catheter and are confronted with the decision as to where to place the drainage bag. Ask yourself *what* questions. "*What* will happen if I place the drainage bag on the bed frame?" The answer could be, "Urine will flow into the drainage bag by gravity." "*What* will happen if I place the drainage bag on an IV pole?" The answer could be, "Urine will remain in the bladder because the IV pole is above the level of the bladder and fluid does not flow uphill, and if there is urine in the bag, it will flow back into the bladder."
- When palpating a pulse you should use gentle compression. Ask yourself the question, "*Why* should I use gentle compression?" The answer could be, "Gentle compression allows you to feel the pulsation of the artery and prevents excessive pressure on the artery that will cut off circulation and thus obliterate the pulse."
- The textbook says that in emergencies nurses should always assess the airway first. Immediately ask, "*Why* should I assess the airway first?" There may be a variety of answers. "In an emergency, follow the ABCs (Airway, Breathing, and Circulation) of assessment, which always begin with the airway. Maslow's Hierarchy of Needs identifies that physiological needs should be met first. Because an airway is essential for the passage of life-sustaining gases in and out of the lungs, this is the priority." Although all of these responses answer the question *why,* only the last answer really provides an in-depth

answer to the *why* question. If your response to the original *why* question raises another *why* question, you need to delve deeper. "*Why* do the ABCs of assessment begin with the airway?" "*Why* should physiological needs be met first?"

- When talking with a patient about an emotionally charged topic, the patient begins to cry. You are confronted with a variety of potential responses. Use the method of *if . . . then* statements. *If . . . then* thinking links an action to a consequence. For example, *if* I remain silent, *then* the patient may refocus on what was said. *If* I say, "You seem very sad," *then* the patient may discuss the feelings being felt at the time. *If* I respond with an open-ended statement, *then* the patient may pursue the topic in relation to individualized concerns. After you explore a variety of courses of action with the *if . . . then* method, you should be in a better position to choose the most appropriate intervention for the situation.
- You will recognize that you have arrived at a more advanced level of critical thinking when determining that your next course of action is based on the concept of *it depends*. For example, a patient suddenly becomes extremely short of breath and you decide to administer oxygen during this emergency. When considering the amount and route of delivery of the oxygen, you recognize that *it depends*. You need to collect more data. You need to ask more questions, such as, "Is the patient already receiving oxygen? Does the patient have a chronic obstructive pulmonary disease? Is the patient a mouth breather? What other signs and symptoms are identified?" The answers to these questions will influence your choice of interventions.

When exploring the *how*, *what*, *where*, *when*, *why*, *if . . . then*, and *it depends* methods of inquiry, you are more likely to arrive at appropriate inferences, assumptions, and conclusions that will ensure effective nursing care.

These same techniques of inquiry can be used when practicing test taking. Reviewing questions that have rationales is an excellent way to explore the reasons for correct and incorrect answers. When answering a question, state why you think your choice is the correct answer and why you think each of the other options is an incorrect answer. This encourages you to focus on the reasons why you responded in a certain way in a particular situation. It prevents you from making quick judgments before exploring the rationales for your actions. After you have done this, compare your rationales with the rationales for the correct and incorrect answers that are provided. Are your rationales focused, methodical, deliberate, logical, relevant, accurate, precise, clear, comprehensive, creative, and reflective? This method of studying not only reviews nursing content but also fosters critical thinking and applies critical thinking to test taking.

During or after the review of an examination, these techniques of inquiry also can be employed, particularly with those questions you got wrong. Although you can conduct this review independently, it is more valuable to review test questions in a group. Your peers and the instructor are valuable resources you should use to facilitate your learning. Different perspectives, experiential backgrounds, and levels of expertise can enhance your inquiry. Be inquisitive. *If you don't go there, you'll never get anywhere.*

OVERCOME BARRIERS TO BEING INQUISITIVE

Effective inquiry requires more than just a simplistic, cursory review of a topic. Therefore, critical thinkers must have curiosity, perseverance, and motivation. **Curiosity** is the desire to learn or know and is a requirement to delve deeper into a topic. If you are uninterested in or apathetic about a topic, you are not going to go that extra mile. Sometimes you may have to "psych yourself up" to study a particular topic. Students frequently say they are overwhelmed by topics such as fluids and electrolytes, blood gases, or chest tubes. As a result, they develop a minimal understanding of these topics and are willing to learn by trial and error in the clinical area or surrender several questions on an examination. Never be willing to let a lack of knowledge be the norm, because this results in incompetence and an unsafe nursing care provider. Overcome this attitude by maximizing your perseverance.

Perseverance means willingness to continue in some effort or course of action despite difficulty or opposition. Critical thinkers never give up until they obtain the information that satisfies their curiosity. To perform a comprehensive inquiry when studying requires time. Make a schedule for studying at the beginning of the week and adhere to it. This prevents procrastination later in the week when you may prefer to rationalize doing something else and postpone studying. In addition, studying 1 hour a day is more effective than studying 7 hours in 1 day. Breaks between study periods allow for the processing of information, and they provide time to rest and regain focus and concentration. The greatest barrier to perseverance is a deadline. When working under a time limit you may not have enough time to process and understand information. The length of time to study for a test depends on the amount and type of content to be tested and how much previous studying has been done. If you study 2 hours every day for 2 weeks during a unit of instruction, a 1-hour review may be adequate for an examination addressing this content. If you are preparing for a comprehensive examination for a course at the end of the semester, you may decide to study 3 hours a night for 1 to 2 weeks. If you are studying for a National Council Licensure Examination (NCLEX), you may decide to study 2 hours a day for 3 months. Only you can determine how much time you need to study or prepare for a test. Perseverance can be enhanced by the use of motivation strategies.

Motivation strategies inspire, prompt, encourage, or instigate you to act. For example, divide the information to be learned into segments and set multiple short-term goals for studying. Cross a segment off the list after you reach a goal. Also, this is the time to use incentives. Reward yourself after an hour of studying. Think about how proud you will be when you earn an excellent grade on the examination. Visualize yourself walking down the aisle at graduation or working as a nurse during your career. Incentives can be more tangible (e.g., eating a snack, reading a book for 10 minutes, playing with a child, or doing anything that strikes your fancy). You should identify the best pattern of studying that satisfies your needs; use motivation techniques to increase your enthusiasm, and then draw on your determination to explore in depth the *how*, *what*, *where*, *when*, and *whys*, *if . . . then*, and *it depends* of nursing practice.

Be Creative: You Must Think Outside the Box!

Creative people are imaginative, inventive, innovative, resourceful, original, and visionary. To find solutions beyond common, predictable, and standardized procedures or practices, you must be creative. Creativity is what allows you to be yourself and individualize the nursing care you provide to each patient. With the explosion of information and technology, the importance of thinking creatively will increase in the future because the "old" ways of doing things will be inadequate. No two situations or two people are ever alike. Therefore, *you must think outside the box!*

OVERCOME BARRIERS TO CREATIVITY

To be creative you must be open-minded, have independence of thought, and be a risk taker. It is difficult to think outside the box when you are not willing to color outside the lines! Being **open-minded** requires you to consider a wide range of ideas, concepts, and opinions before framing an opinion or making judgments. You must identify your opinions, beliefs, biases, stereotypes, and prejudices. We all have them to one extent or another, so do not deny them. However, they must be recognized, compartmentalized, and not imposed on patients. Unless these attitudes are placed in perspective, they will interfere with critical thinking. In every situation you need to remain open to all perspectives, not just your own. When you think that your opinion is the only right opinion, you are engaging in egocentric thinking. *Egocentric thinking* is based on the belief that the world exists or can be known only in relation to the individual's mind. This rigid thinking creates a barrier around your brain that obstructs the inflow of information, imaginative thinking, and the outflow of innovative ideas. An example of an instance in which you have been open-minded is one in which you have changed your mind after having had a discussion with someone else. The new information convinced you to think outside of your original thoughts and opinions.

Independence of thought means the ability to consider all the possibilities and then arrive at an autonomous conclusion. To do this you need to feel comfortable with ambiguity. *Ambiguous* means having two or more meanings and is therefore being uncertain, unclear, indefinite, and vague. For example, a nursing student may be taught by an instructor to establish a sterile field for a sterile dressing change by using the inside of the package of the sterile gloves. When following a sterile dressing change procedure in a clinical skills book, the directions may state to use a separate sterile cloth for the sterile field. When practicing this procedure with another student, the other student may open several 4 × 4 gauze packages and leave them open as their sterile fields. As a beginning nursing student, this is difficult to understand because of a limited relevant knowledge base and experiential background. Frequently, thinking is concrete and follows rules and procedures, is black and white, or is correct or incorrect. It takes knowledge and experience to recognize that you have many options and may still follow the principles of sterile technique. Remember, "There is more than one road to Rome!"

To travel a different path requires taking risks. *Risk* in the dictionary means the chance of injury, damage, or loss. However, **risk taking** in relation to nursing refers to considering all the options, eliminating potential danger to a patient, and acting in a reasoned, logical, and safe manner when implementing unique interventions. Being creative requires intellectual stamina and a willingness to go where no one has been before. Risk takers tend to be leaders, not followers. The greatest personal risk of creativity is the blow to the ego when confronted with failure. However, you must recognize that throughout your nursing career you will be faced with outcomes that are successful as well as those that are unsuccessful. How you manage your feelings with regard to each, particularly those that are unsuccessful, will influence your willingness to take future creative risks. Successful outcomes build confidence. Unsuccessful outcomes should not be defeating or prevent future creativity when appropriately examined. The whole purpose of evaluation in the nursing process is to compare and contrast patient outcomes with expected outcomes. If expected outcomes are not attained, the entire process must be re-examined and then re-performed. You must recognize that:

- Unsuccessful outcomes do occur.
- Unsuccessful outcomes may not be a reflection of your competence.
- The number of successful outcomes far outnumbers the number of unsuccessful outcomes.

When you accept these facts, then you may feel more confident to take risks with your creativity.

CRITICAL THINKING APPLIED TO TEST TAKING

Educational Domains

Nursing as a discipline includes three domains of learning—affective, psychomotor, and cognitive. The **affective domain** is concerned with attitudes, values, and the development of appreciations. An example of nursing care in the affective domain is the nurse quietly accepting a patient's statement that there is no God without the nurse imposing personal beliefs on the patient. The **psychomotor domain** is concerned with manipulative or motor skills related to procedures or physical interventions. An example of nursing care in the psychomotor domain is the nurse administering an intramuscular injection to a patient. The **cognitive domain** is concerned with recall, recognition of knowledge, comprehension, and the development and application of intellectual skills and abilities. An example of nursing care in the cognitive domain is the nurse clustering collected information and determining its significance.

Components of a Multiple-Choice Question

A multiple-choice question is called an **item.** Each item has two parts. The **stem** is the part that contains the information that identifies the topic and its parameters and then asks a question or forms the beginning portion of a sentence that is completed by the correct option. The second part consists of one or more possible responses, which are called **options.** One of the options is the correct answer, and the others are wrong answers (also called **distractors**).

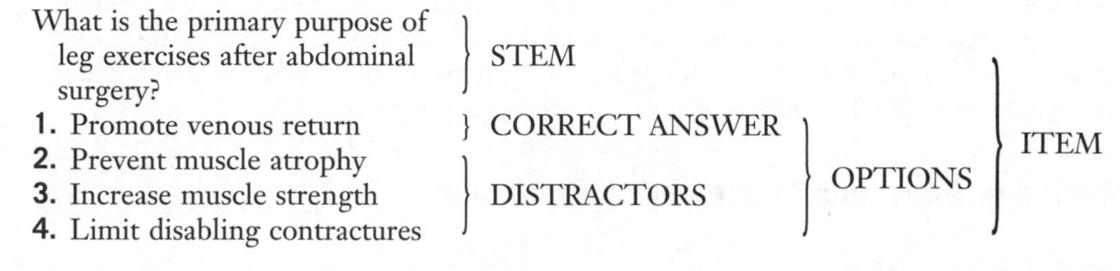

Cognitive Levels of Nursing Questions

Questions on nursing examinations reflect a variety of thinking processes that nurses use when caring for patients. These thinking processes are part of the cognitive domain and they progress from the simple to the complex, from the concrete to the abstract, and from the tangible to the intangible. There are four major types of thinking processes represented by nursing questions:

- **Knowledge Questions,** in which the emphasis is on recalling remembered information.
- **Comprehension Questions,** in which the emphasis is on understanding the meaning and intent of remembered information.
- **Application Questions,** in which the emphasis is on remembering understood information and utilizing the information in new situations.
- **Analysis Questions,** in which the emphasis is on comparing and contrasting a variety of elements of information.

CRITICAL-THINKING STRATEGY TO ANSWER NURSING QUESTIONS: THE RACE MODEL

Answering a test question is like participating in a race. Of course, you want to come in first and be the winner. However, the thing to remember about a race is that success is based not just on speed but also on strategy and tactics. The same is true about success on nursing examinations. Although speed may be a variable that must be considered when taking a timed test so that the amount of time spent on each question is factored into the test strategy, the emphasis should be on the use of critical-thinking strategies to answer test questions. The RACE model presented here is a critical-thinking strategy to use when answering nursing questions. If you follow the RACE model every time you examine a test question, its use will become second nature. This methodical approach will improve your abilities to analyze a test question critically and will improve your chances of selecting the correct answer.

The RACE model has four steps to answering a test question:

R *R*ecognizc kcywords.

A *A*sk what the question is asking.

C *C*ritically analyze each option in relation to the question and the other options.
- *C*ritically scrutinize each option in relation to the information in the stem.
- *C*ritically identify a rationale for each option.
- *C*ritically compare and contrast the options in relation to the information in the stem and their relationships with one another.

E *E*liminate incorrect options.
- *E*liminate one option at a time.
- *E*liminate as many incorrect options as possible.

The following discussion explores this critical-thinking strategy in relation to the thinking processes represented in nursing test questions. Thoughtfully read the *Cognitive Requirements* under each type of question (e.g., Knowledge, Comprehension, Application, and Analysis). It is important to understand this content to apply the critical-thinking strategies inherent in each cognitive-level question. In addition, three sets of sample test questions are presented to demonstrate the increasing complexity of thinking reflected in the various cognitive levels focusing on specific fundamentals of nursing content. Also, each cognitive level includes the RACE model applied to an alternate-type item.

Knowledge Questions: Remember Information!

COGNITIVE REQUIREMENTS

Knowledge is information that is filed or stored in the brain. It represents the elements essential to the core of a discipline. In nursing, this information consists of elements such as terminology and specific facts including steps of procedures, phenomena, expected laboratory values, classifications, and the expected ranges of vital signs. This type of information requires no alteration from one use or application to another because it is concrete. The information is recalled or recognized in the form in which it was originally learned. This information is the foundation of critical thinking. You must have adequate, accurate, relevant, and important information on which to base your more theoretical, abstract thinking.

Beginning nursing students find knowledge-level questions the easiest because they require the recall or regurgitation of information. Information may be memorized, which involves repeatedly reviewing information to place it and keep it in the brain. Information also can be committed to memory through repeated experiences with the information. Repetition is necessary because information is forgotten quickly unless reinforced. When answering knowledge-level questions you either know the information or you don't. The challenge of answering knowledge-level questions is defining what the question is asking and tapping your knowledge. See our textbook *TEST SUCCESS: Test-Taking Techniques for Beginning Nursing Students* (F.A. Davis) for specific study techniques related to knowledge-level questions.

USE THE RACE MODEL TO ANSWER KNOWLEDGE-LEVEL QUESTIONS

1. Which is the classification of the medication docusate sodium?
1. Stool softener
2. Cardiac glycoside
3. Histamine H_2 antagonist
4. Calcium channel blocker

IMPLEMENT THE RACE MODEL: A CRITICAL-THINKING STRATEGY

Recognize keywords.	Which is the **classification** of the medication **docusate sodium**?
Ask what the question is asking.	What category of medication is docusate sodium?
Critically analyze each option in relation to the question and the other options.	This question does not require complex understanding, comparative analysis, or application skills; it requires only recall of information about docusate sodium. **Rationales:** **1. Stool softeners are medications that promote the elimination of fecal material. Docusate sodium is a stool softener.** **2.** Cardiac glycosides increase cardiac output by decreasing the heart rate and strengthening cardiac contractions. Docusate sodium is not a cardiac glycoside.

	3. Histamine-2 (H_2) antagonists are medications that inhibit histamine at H_2 sites in the parietal cells in the stomach, which reduces gastric acid secretion. Docusate sodium is not an H_2 antagonist. **4.** Calcium channel blockers are medications that inhibit calcium ion influx across cell membranes during cardiac depolarization. They dilate coronary and peripheral arteries, relax coronary vascular smooth muscles, and slow sinoatrial/atrioventricular node conduction time. Docusate sodium is not a calcium channel blocker.
Eliminate incorrect options.	Because options 2, 3, and 4 are not the names of the classification of docusate sodium, they can be eliminated. If you know the action of one or more of the incorrect options it may help you eliminate them.

2. Which is the description of the interviewing technique of paraphrasing?
1. Asking the patient to repeat what was just said
2. Condensing a discussion into an organized review
3. Restating what the patient has said using similar words
4. Asking goal-directed questions concentrating on key concerns

IMPLEMENT THE RACE MODEL: A CRITICAL-THINKING STRATEGY

Recognize keywords.	Which is the **description** of the interviewing technique of **paraphrasing**?
Ask what the question is asking.	How is the interviewing technique of paraphrasing implemented?
Critically analyze each option in relation to the question and the other options.	To answer this question you must know the definition or characteristic of paraphrasing. It is information that you must recall from your memory. You do not have to know other interviewing skills or their descriptions and characteristics to answer this question correctly. **Rationales:** **1.** Asking a patient to repeat what was just asked is known as clarifying, not paraphrasing. **2.** Reviewing a discussion is known as summarizing, not paraphrasing. **3. Paraphrasing or restating is an interviewing skill in which the nurse listens for a patient's basic message and then repeats the contents of the message in similar words. This validates information from the patient without changing the meaning of the statement and provides an opportunity for the patient to hear what was said.** **4.** Asking goal-directed questions that concentrate on key concerns is known as focusing, not paraphrasing.
Eliminate incorrect options.	Options 1, 2, and 4 are not examples of paraphrasing and can be eliminated. Although you do not have to know the characteristics of interviewing skills other than paraphrasing to answer this question correctly, knowing this information may help you eliminate incorrect options.

3. What is another name for a decubitus ulcer?
1. Skin tear
2. Pressure ulcer
3. Surface abrasion
4. Penetrating wound

IMPLEMENT THE RACE MODEL: A CRITICAL-THINKING STRATEGY

Recognize keywords.	What is **another name** for a **decubitus ulcer**?
Ask what the question is asking.	What is an alternate name for a decubitus ulcer?
Critically analyze each option in relation to the question and the other options.	To answer this question you must know the alternate name for a decubitus ulcer. It is information you must recollect from your memory. You do not have to know the description or characteristics of other types of wounds to answer this question. **Rationales:** 1. A skin tear is a break in the continuity of thin, fragile skin caused by friction or shearing force. 2. **A pressure ulcer is impaired skin (reddened area, sore, or lesion characterized by sloughing of tissue) over a bony prominence caused by pressure that interferes with the delivery of oxygen to body cells.** 3. An abrasion is the scraping or rubbing away of the superficial layers of the skin. 4. A penetrating wound occurs when a sharp object pierces the skin and injures underlying tissues.
Eliminate incorrect options.	Options 1, 3, and 4 are not other names for a decubitus ulcer and can be eliminated. Although it is not necessary to know the description and characteristics of other types of wounds to answer the question correctly, knowing this information may help you eliminate incorrect options.

4. Which is the name of this type of syringe?
   1. Insulin
   2. Irrigation
   3. Intradermal
   4. Subcutaneous

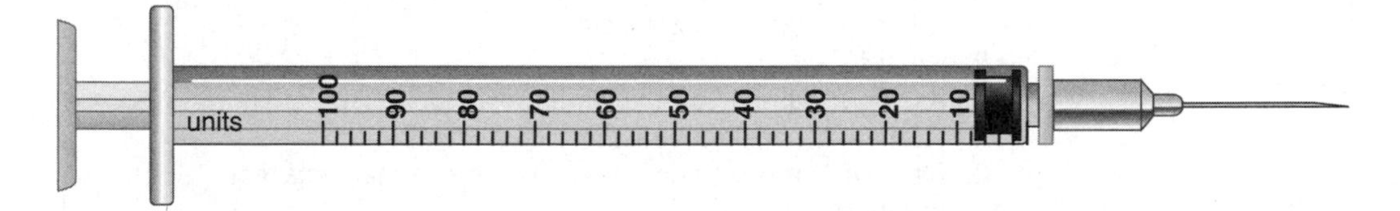

IMPLEMENT THE RACE MODEL: A CRITICAL-THINKING STRATEGY

Recognize keywords.	Which is the **name** of this type of **syringe**?
Ask what the question is asking.	Identify the name of the type of syringe that is marked in units depicted in the illustration?
Critically analyze each option in relation to the question and the other options.	To answer this question you must identify that the syringe in the illustration is an insulin syringe. This question does not require complex understanding, comparative analysis, or application skills; it requires only recall of the name of this type of syringe. **Rationales:** 1. **This is an illustration of an insulin syringe. It is a U-100 syringe marked in units, of which there are 100 units per mL.** 2. This is not an illustration of a syringe used for irrigating a wound. Generally a piston syringe that can contain up to 50 mL of solution is used to irrigate a wound; it has a tip to which a catheter can be attached.

	3. This is not an illustration of a syringe used to administer a medication via the intradermal route. Generally a 1-mL tuberculin syringe marked in 0.01 mL (1/100th of a milliliter) and minims (16 minims is equal to 1 mL) is used to administer a medication via the intradermal route. **4.** This is not an illustration of a syringe that is used to administer a medication via the subcutaneous route. Generally a 3-mL standard syringe marked in whole milliliters and 0.1 mL (1/10th of a milliliter) with a ⅝-, ½-, or 1-inch length needle is used to administer a medication into subcutaneous tissue.
Eliminate incorrect options.	Because options 2, 3, and 4 are not the names of the type of syringe depicted in the illustration, they can be eliminated.

Comprehension Questions: Understand Information!

COGNITIVE REQUIREMENTS

Comprehension is the ability to understand that which is known. To be safe practitioners, nurses must understand information such as reasons for nursing interventions, physiology and pathophysiology, consequences of actions, and responses to medications. To reach an understanding of information in nursing you must be able to translate information into your own words to personalize its meaning. Once information is rearranged in your own mind, you must interpret the essential components for their intent, corollaries, significance, implications, consequences, and conclusions in accordance with the conditions described in the original communication. The information is manipulated within its own context without being used in a different or new situation.

Beginning nursing students generally consider comprehension-level questions slightly more difficult than knowledge-level questions but less complicated than application-level and analysis-level questions. Students often try to deal with comprehension-level information by memorizing the content. For example, when studying local signs and symptoms of an infection, students may memorize the following list: heat, erythema, pain, edema, and exudate. Although this can be done, it is far better to understand why these adaptations occur. Erythema and heat occur because of increased circulation to the area. Edema occurs because of increased permeability of the capillaries. Pain occurs because the accumulating fluid in the tissue presses on nerve endings. Exudate occurs because of the accumulation of fluid, cells, and other substances at the site of infection. The mind is a wonderful machine, but unless you have a photographic memory, lists of information without understanding often become overwhelming and confusing. The challenge of answering comprehension questions is to understand the information. See our textbook *TEST SUCCESS: Test-Taking Techniques for Beginning Nursing Students* for specific study techniques related to comprehension-level questions.

USE THE RACE MODEL TO ANSWER COMPREHENSION-LEVEL QUESTIONS

1. How does the medication docusate sodium facilitate defecation?
   1. Softens stool
   2. Forms a bulk residue
   3. Irritates the intestinal wall
   4. Dilates the intestinal lumen

IMPLEMENT THE RACE MODEL: A CRITICAL-THINKING STRATEGY

Recognize keywords.	**How** does the medication **docusate sodium facilitate defecation**?
Ask what the question is asking.	How does docusate sodium work in the body to promote the passage of stool?
Critically analyze each option in relation to the question and to the other options.	The word in the stem that indicates this is a comprehension-level question is *facilitate*. You should scrutinize each option to identify whether the description in the option correctly explains how or why docusate sodium works to facilitate defecation. **Rationales:** 1. **Docusate sodium softens and delays the drying of feces by lowering the surface tension of water, permitting water and fat to penetrate the feces.** 2. Bulk-forming laxatives, such as psyllium hydrophilic mucilloid, increase the fluid, gaseous, or solid bulk in the intestines. 3. Irritants or stimulants, such as bisacodyl, irritate the intestinal mucosa or stimulate intestinal wall nerve endings, which precipitates peristalsis. 4. Large-volume enemas, not medications, enlarge the lumen of the intestine, which precipitates peristalsis.
Eliminate incorrect options.	Options 2, 3, and 4 do not accurately describe the therapeutic action of docusate sodium and can be eliminated. You do not have to know the therapeutic action of other medications that facilitate defecation to answer the question correctly. However, this information may help you eliminate incorrect options.

2. How does the interviewing technique of paraphrasing promote communication?
   1. Requires patients to defend their points of view
   2. Limits patients from continuing a rambling conversation
   3. Allows patients to take their conversations in any desired direction
   4. Offers patients an opportunity to develop a clearer idea of what they said

IMPLEMENT THE RACE MODEL: A CRITICAL-THINKING STRATEGY

Recognize keywords.	**How** does the interviewing technique of **paraphrasing promote communication**?
Ask what the question is asking.	How does paraphrasing encourage communication?
Critically analyze each option in relation to the question and to the other options.	The word in the stem that indicates that this is a comprehension-level question is *promote*. You should scrutinize each option to identify whether the description in the option correctly explains the consequence of using paraphrasing as a communication technique. **Rationales:** 1. Requiring patients to defend their points of view describes the results of challenging statements that usually are barriers to communication. 2. Limiting patients from continuing a rambling conversation describes one purpose of the interviewing skill of focusing, which is the use of questions or statements to center on one concern mentioned within a wordy, confusing conversation. 3. Allowing patients to take their conversations in any desired direction is the purpose of open-ended questions or statements.

	4. Paraphrasing involves actively listening for the patient's concerns, which are then restated by the nurse in similar words. This intervention conveys that the nurse has heard and understood the message and gives the patient an opportunity to review what was said.
Eliminate incorrect options.	Options 1, 2, and 3 do not accurately describe how paraphrasing works to promote communication and can be eliminated. You do not have to know how other interviewing skills work to facilitate communication to answer the question correctly. However, this information may help you eliminate incorrect options.

3. How does turning patients every 2 hours prevent pressure ulcers from developing?
1. Relieves weight on the capillaries, allowing oxygen to reach body cells
2. Promotes muscle contractions, increasing the basal metabolic rate of the body
3. Keeps the extremities dependent, permitting blood to flow to distal cells by gravity
4. Drops the organs in the abdominal cavity by gravity, relieving pressure against the diaphragm

IMPLEMENT THE RACE MODEL: A CRITICAL-THINKING STRATEGY

Recognize keywords.	**How** does **turning** patients every 2 hours **prevent pressure ulcers** from developing?
Ask what the question is asking.	How does turning a patient prevent decubitus ulcers?
Critically analyze each option in relation to the question and to the other options.	The word in the stem that indicates that this is a comprehension-level question is *prevent.* You should scrutinize each option to identify whether the description in the option correctly explains how turning a patient relieves pressure and prevents a pressure ulcer. **Rationales:** **1. Capillary beds are compressed and blood flow is obliterated with excessive external pressure (12 to 32 mm Hg). Changing position removes the weight of the body off dependent areas, permitting blood to flow through the capillaries, thus supporting gaseous exchange at the cellular level.** **2.** Muscle contraction expends energy that raises the basal metabolic rate; however, this is unrelated to the development of pressure ulcers. **3.** Blood flow to the extremities increases when the extremities are kept below the level of the heart; however, this is unrelated to the development of pressure ulcers. **4.** Relieving pressure against the diaphragm by abdominal organs allows for greater thoracic expansion; however, this is unrelated to the development of pressure ulcers.
Eliminate incorrect options.	Options 2, 3, and 4 do not accurately explain how turning relieves pressure, thereby preventing a pressure ulcer, and can be eliminated. Understanding the concept of gravity in relation to options 3 and 4 may help you eliminate these options because they are unrelated to pressure ulcer development.

4. Which is the purpose of administering a medication using a 45° angle and 1½-inch needle length as indicated in the illustration?
1. Injects medication via the intramuscular route
2. Injects medication via the subcutaneous route
3. Injects medication via the intravascular route
4. Injects medication via the intradermal route

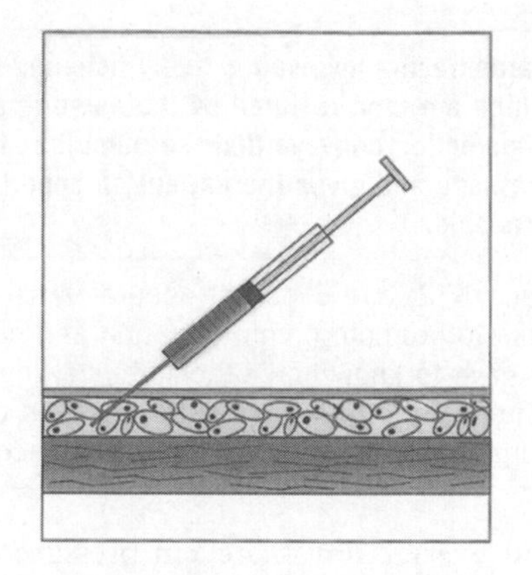

IMPLEMENT THE RACE MODEL: A CRITICAL-THINKING STRATEGY

Recognize keywords.	Which is the **purpose of administering** a medication using a 45° angle and 1½-inch needle length **as indicated in the illustration**?
Ask what the question is asking.	Which route of administration is performed when an injection is given using a 1½-needle at a 45° angle?
Critically analyze each option in relation to the question and to the other options.	To answer this question you must know that when using a 1½-inch length needle at a 45° angle medication is injected into subcutaneous tissue. **Rationale:** **1.** A muscle is not accessed via a 45° angle using a 1½-inch needle. A 90° angle of insertion is standard for administering medication via the intramuscular route. A muscle is below the level of subcutaneous tissue. A needle length of 1½ inches is necessary to reach muscle tissue in most adults, a 2-inch length needle is used to administer an intramuscular injection to an obese adult, and a 1-inch needle length is used when administering an intramuscular injection in the deltoid muscle. **2. This is an illustration of a medication injected via the subcutaneous route. A syringe with a 1½-inch needle inserted at a 45° angle ensures that medication is injected into subcutaneous tissue and not into a muscle.** **3.** A vein is not accessed via a 45° angle using a 1½-inch needle. The intravascular route requires administration of a medication directly into a vein. This can be accomplished by adding medication to a large-volume bag of intravenous fluid, a single dose of medication mixed with a small volume of fluid in its own intravenous bag via secondary tubing attached to a current primary intravenous line (Piggbyback) or via a Bolus (push) single dose of medication inserted directly into a primary line or venous access device. **4.** Below the epidermis is not accessed via a 45° angle using a 1½-inch needle. A 15° angle of insertion is used to administer medication via the intradermal route.
Eliminate incorrect options.	Options 1, 3, and 4 can be eliminated because these routes inject medication into areas of the body other than subcutaneous tissue that is depicted in the illustration. If you know the names of the routes that require other than a 45° angle of insertion such as option 1 (intramuscular 90° angle) or option 3 (intradermal 15° angle), you can eliminate these 2 options from consideration, thereby increasing your chances of selecting the correct answer.

Application Questions: Use Information!

COGNITIVE REQUIREMENTS

Application is the ability to use known and understood information in new situations. It requires more than just understanding information because you must demonstrate, solve, change, modify, or manipulate information in other than its originally learned form or context. With application questions you are confronted with a new situation that requires you to recall information and manipulate the information from within a familiar context to arrive at abstractions, generalizations, or consequences regarding the information that can be used in the new situation to answer the question. Application questions require you to make rational, logical judgments.

Beginning nursing students frequently find these questions challenging because they require a restructuring of understood information into abstractions, commonalities, and generalizations, which are then applied to new situations. You do this all the time. Although there are parts of your day that are routine, every day you are exposed to new, challenging experiences. The same concept holds true for application questions. With application questions you will be confronted by situations that you learned about in a book, experienced personally, relived through other students' experiences, or never heard about or experienced before. This will happen throughout your entire nursing career. The challenge of answering application questions is going beyond rules and regulations and using information in a unique, creative way. See our textbook *TEST SUCCESS: Test-Taking Techniques for Beginning Nursing Students* for specific study techniques related to application-level questions.

USE THE RACE MODEL TO ANSWER APPLICATION-LEVEL QUESTIONS

1. A patient complains about not having had a bowel movement in 3 days. Which classification of drugs is helpful in relieving this problem?
   1. Stool softener
   2. Cardiac glycoside
   3. Histamine H_2 antagonist
   4. Calcium channel blocker

IMPLEMENT THE RACE MODEL: A CRITICAL-THINKING STRATEGY

Recognize keywords.	A patient complains about **not having had a bowel movement** in 3 days. Which **classification** of **drugs** is **helpful** in **relieving** this problem?
Ask what the question is asking.	Which classification of drugs is most helpful in facilitating defecation, thus relieving constipation?
Critically analyze each option in relation to the question and to the other options.	The words in the stem that indicate that this is an application question are *helpful in relieving.* To choose which classification of drugs will be most helpful in relieving this patient's problem, you must know that a patient who has not had a bowel movement in 3 days may be constipated, the therapeutic action and outcome of various classifications of drugs, and which classification of drugs would be helpful in relieving constipation. **Rationales:** 1. **Docusate sodium is a stool softener. It increases water and fat penetration of feces, which softens the stool.** 2. Cardiac glycosides increase the force of cardiac contractions, which increases the cardiac output (positive inotropic effect), and decrease electrical conduction in the heart, which decreases the heart rate (positive dromotropic effect). Docusate sodium is not a cardiac glycoside.

continued

continued

	3. Histamine-2 (H_2) antagonists inhibit histamine at H_2 receptor sites in parietal cells, and this inhibits gastric acid secretion. Docusate sodium is not an H_2 antagonist. **4.** Calcium channel blockers inhibit calcium ion influx across cell membranes during cardiac depolarization. They relax coronary vascular smooth muscles, dilate coronary and peripheral arteries, and slow sinoatrial/atrioventricular node conduction times. Docusate sodium is not a calcium channel blocker.
Eliminate incorrect options.	Because options 2, 3, and 4 are unrelated to facilitating the passage of stool, they can be eliminated. You do not have to know the expected outcome of the drug classifications in the incorrect options to answer the question correctly. However, if you know this information it may help you eliminate these options.

2. A patient scheduled for major surgery, who is perspiring and nervously picking at the bed linen, says, "I don't know if I can go through with this surgery." The nurse responds, "You'd rather not have surgery now?" Which interviewing technique was used by the nurse?

1. Focusing
2. Reflection
3. Paraphrasing
4. Clarification

IMPLEMENT THE RACE MODEL: A CRITICAL-THINKING STRATEGY

Recognize keywords.	A patient scheduled for major surgery, who is perspiring and nervously picking at the bed linen, says, "I don't know if I can go through with this surgery." The nurse responds, **"You'd rather not have surgery now?" Which** interviewing **technique was used** by the nurse?
Ask what the question is asking.	What interviewing technique is being used by the nurse when the nurse says in response to the patient, "You'd rather not have surgery now?"
Critically analyze each option in relation to the question and to the other options.	The words in the stem that indicate that this is an application question are *was used.* To identify which technique was used by the nurse you have to understand the elements of a paraphrasing statement and you must recognize a paraphrasing statement when it is used. **Rationales:** **1.** The example in the stem is not using focusing because the patient's statement was short and contained one message that was reiterated by the nurse. Focusing is used to explore one concern among many statements made by the patient. **2.** The example in the stem is not using reflection because the nurse's statement is concerned with the content, not the underlying feeling, of the patient's statement. An example of reflection used by the nurse is, "You seem anxious about having major surgery." **3. The nurse used paraphrasing because the patient's and nurse's statements contain the same message but they are expressed with different words.** **4.** The example in the stem is not using clarification. When clarification is used, the nurse is asking the patient to further explain what is meant by the patient's statement. An example of clarification used by the nurse is, "I am not quite sure that I know what you mean when you say you would rather not have surgery now."

Eliminate incorrect options.	Options 1, 2, and 4 can be eliminated because these techniques are different from the technique portrayed in the nurse's response in the stem. Although it is helpful to understand the elements of the other interviewing techniques because it will help you eliminate incorrect options, it is not necessary to understand this information to answer the question correctly.

3. A nurse identifies that a patient on prolonged bed rest may be developing a pressure ulcer. Which color of the skin over a bony prominence supports this conclusion?

1. Red
2. Blue
3. Black
4. Yellow

IMPLEMENT THE RACE MODEL: A CRITICAL-THINKING STRATEGY

Recognize keywords.	A nurse identifies that a patient may be developing a **pressure ulcer. Which color of** the **skin** over a **bony prominence** supports this conclusion?
Ask what the question is asking.	Which early sign indicates a pressure ulcer over a bony prominence?
Critically analyze each option in relation to the question and to the other options.	The words in the stem that indicate that this is an application question are *identifies* and *developing a pressure ulcer.* To answer this question you have to understand how and why pressure can cause a pressure ulcer and know the common early sign that indicates the formation of a pressure ulcer. **Rationales:** **1. Erythema is a red discoloration generally caused by local vasodilation in an attempt to bring more oxygen to the area.** **2.** Cyanosis is a bluish color caused by an increased amount of deoxygenated hemoglobin associated with hypoxia, not pressure. **3.** Eschar generally appears black and is the scab or dry crust that results from death of tissue. **4.** Jaundice is a yellow-orange color caused by increased deposits of bilirubin in tissue, not a response to pressure.
Eliminate incorrect options.	Options 2, 3, and 4 are not early signs of a pressure ulcer and are incorrect answers. Although it is helpful to know what is happening when the skin reflects each of the colors indicated in the options so that you can eliminate incorrect answers, it is not necessary to know this information to answer the question.

4. A patient has a prescription for regular insulin coverage before meals. The prescription states to administer regular insulin based on blood glucose results.

150 to 175 mg/dL: 2 units
176 to 225 mg/dL: 4 units
226 to 275 mg/dL: 6 units
276 mg/dL or more: notify primary health-care provider

The patient's blood glucose level before breakfast is 177 mg/dL. How many units of regular insulin should the nurse administer? **Record your answer using a whole number.**

Answer: __________units

IMPLEMENT THE RACE MODEL: A CRITICAL-THINKING STRATEGY

Recognize keywords.	A patient has a prescription for regular insulin coverage before meals. The prescription states to administer regular insulin based on blood glucose results. **150 to 175 mg/dL: 2 units** **176 to 225 mg/dL: 4 units** **226 to 275 mg/dL: 6 units** **276 mg/dL or more: notify primary health-care provider** The patient's blood glucose level before breakfast is **177 mg/dL. How many units of regular insulin should the nurse administer**? Record your answer using a whole number. Answer: ________Units
Ask what the question is asking.	How many units of regular insulin should the nurse administer when the patient's blood glucose level is 177 mg/dL?
Critically analyze each option in relation to the question and to the other options.	A fill-in-the-blank question does not have several options within the question. Generally you have to insert the information contained in the question into a mathematical formula to manipulate the information to arrive at an answer. However, this fill-in-the-blank item does not require a formula to answer the question. You have to compare the patient's glucose level of 177 mg/dL with the regular insulin prescription to arrive at the correct answer. **Rationale:** **The patient's glucose level is 177 mg/dL. The prescription for regular insulin indicates that if the patient's glucose level is 176 to 225 mg/dL the patient should receive 4 units of regular insulin.**
Eliminate incorrect options.	Because the patient's glucose level is 177 mg/dL the other parameters for glucose levels and their accompanying regular insulin doses can be eliminated.

Analysis Questions: Scrutinize Information!

COGNITIVE REQUIREMENTS

Analysis is the separation of an entity into its constituent parts and examination of their essential features in relation to each other. Analysis questions assume that you know, understand, and can apply information. They ask you to engage in higher-level critical-thinking strategies. To answer analysis-level questions, you first must examine each element of information as a separate entity. Second, you need to investigate the differences among the various elements of information. In other words, you must compare and contrast information. Third, you must analyze the structure and organization of the compared and contrasted information to arrive at a conclusion or answer. Analysis questions often ask you to set priorities and in the stem frequently use words such as *first*, *initially*, *best*, *priority*, and *most important*.

Beginning nursing students find analysis-level questions the most difficult to answer. Analysis questions demand scrutiny of individual elements of information as well as require identification of differences among elements of information. Sometimes students cannot identify the structural or organizational relationship of elements of information. The challenge of answering analysis questions is performing a complete scrutiny of all the various elements of information and their interrelationships without overanalyzing or "reading into" the questions. See our textbook *TEST SUCCESS: Test-Taking Techniques for Beginning Nursing Students* for specific study techniques related to analysis-level questions.

USE THE RACE MODEL TO ANSWER ANALYSIS-LEVEL QUESTIONS

1. A frail, malnourished older adult has been experiencing constipation. Which medication does the nurse anticipate that the primary health-care provider will **most** likely prescribe?
1. Bisacodyl
2. Mineral oil
3. Docusate sodium
4. Magnesium hydroxide

IMPLEMENT THE RACE MODEL: A CRITICAL-THINKING STRATEGY

Recognize keywords.	A **frail, malnourished older adult** has been experiencing **constipation.** Which **medication** does the nurse anticipate that the primary health-care provider will **most likely prescribe?**
Ask what the question is asking.	Which medication that promotes defecation is least likely to cause problems in a debilitated older adult?
Critically analyze each option in relation to the question and the other options.	Analysis questions often ask you to set priorities as indicated by the words *most likely prescribe* in the stem of this question. This question requires you to: understand that frail, malnourished older adults have minimal compensatory reserve in various body systems to manage responses to cathartics and laxatives; know the physiological action, outcome, side effects, and toxic effects of all four medications presented in the stem; contrast and compare the drugs and the risks they pose in the older adult to arrive at which drug would be the least risky drug. The least risky drug is the one that is most likely to be prescribed. **Rationales:** **1.** Bisacodyl irritates the intestinal mucosa, stimulates nerve endings in the wall of the intestines, and causes rapid propulsion of waste from the body. Bisacodyl is not the best choice of a laxative for an older adult because it can cause intestinal cramps, fluid and electrolyte imbalances, and irritation of the intestinal mucosa. **2.** Mineral oil lubricates feces in the colon; however, it can inhibit the absorption of fat-soluble vitamins and is not the best laxative for an older adult. **3. Docusate sodium permits fat and water to penetrate feces, which soften stool. Of all the options, docusate sodium has the fewest side effects in older adults.** **4.** Magnesium hydroxide draws water into the intestine by osmosis, which stimulates peristalsis. It is contraindicated for an older adult because it can cause fluid and electrolyte imbalances and inhibit absorption of fat-soluble vitamins.
Eliminate incorrect options.	Options 1, 2, and 4 are more potent than the correct answer and therefore are least likely to be ordered to relieve constipation in a debilitated older adult. Because you must compare and contrast the drugs in the options presented, the more you know about these medications, the more options you may be able to eliminate, increasing your chances of selecting the correct answer.

2. The mother of a terminally ill child says, "I never thought that I would have such a sick child." Which is the **best** initial response by the nurse?
1. "How do you feel right now?"
2. "What do you mean by sick child?"
3. "Life is not fair to do this to a child."
4. "A sick child is something you never expected."

IMPLEMENT THE RACE MODEL: A CRITICAL-THINKING STRATEGY

Recognize keywords.	The mother of a terminally ill child says, "I never thought that I would have such a sick child." What is the **best initial response** by the nurse?
Ask what the question is asking.	Which is an example of the best interviewing skill to use when initially responding to a statement made by the mother of a terminally ill child?
Critically analyze each option in relation to the question and the other options.	Analysis questions often ask you to set priorities as indicated by the words *best initial response* in the stem of this question. To answer this question you need to: identify which interviewing techniques are portrayed in the statements in each option; understand how and why each interviewing skill works; compare and contrast the pros and cons of each technique if used in this situation; and identify which technique is the most supportive, appropriate, and best initial response by the nurse.
	Rationales: 1. Direct questions cut off communication and should be avoided. 2. This response focuses on the seriousness of the child's illness, which is not the issue raised in the mother's statement. 3. This statement reflects the beliefs and values of the nurse, which should be avoided. 4. **This is a declarative statement that paraphrases the mother's comment. It communicates to the mother that the nurse is attentively listening and invites the mother to expand on her thoughts if she feels ready.**
Eliminate incorrect options.	Options 1, 2, and 3 can be eliminated because they do not focus on the content of the mother's statement.

3. Which patient has the greatest risk for developing a pressure ulcer?
   1. An older adult on bed rest
   2. A toddler learning to walk
   3. A thin young woman in a coma
   4. An emotionally unstable middle-aged man

IMPLEMENT THE RACE MODEL: A CRITICAL-THINKING STRATEGY

Recognize keywords.	Which patient has the **greatest risk** for **developing** a **pressure ulcer**?
Ask what the question is asking.	Which patient in the various age groups is at the greatest risk for a pressure ulcer?
Critically analyze each option in relation to the question and to the other options.	Analysis questions often ask you to set priorities as indicated by the words *greatest risk* in the stem of this question. To answer this question you need to know what major risk factors contribute to the development of a pressure ulcer, identify the risk factors for pressure ulcer development in all four of the specific categories of the life span represented in the options, and assign a level of risk to each of the individuals identified in the options in comparison with each of the other individuals. Once you complete this intellectual analysis, you will identify the individual at greatest risk. **Rationales:** 1. Although the skin of older adults is vulnerable to the development of pressure ulcers because of decreased subcutaneous fat, reduced thickness and vascularity of the dermis, and decreased sebaceous gland activity, older adults are still capable of changing position and moving around in bed, which relieves pressure on integumentary tissue.

	2. A toddler learning to walk is not immobile. In addition, the skin of toddlers usually has adequate circulation, subcutaneous tissue, and hydration and is supple. A toddler may fall and develop bruises (contusions) or scrapes (abrasions), not pressure ulcers. **3. Of the options offered, a thin young woman in a coma is the most vulnerable for developing a pressure ulcer. A thin person has little protective subcutaneous fat over bony prominences, and a person in a coma is immobile and unable to move or turn purposefully. Immobility results in prolonged pressure, which interferes with the oxygen supply to body cells.** **4.** Middle-aged men usually do not exhibit the effects of aging on the integumentary system. In addition, emotionally unstable people are able to move and change positions, which permit circulation to the cells of the skin.
Eliminate incorrect options.	Individuals presented in options 1, 2, and 4 are at less of a risk for the development of pressure ulcers than a thin person who is immobile.

4. A patient has a prescription for 20 units of NPH insulin and 6 units of regular insulin to be administered subcutaneously at 0800. Insert an arrow at the line on the barrel of the syringe to where the total insulin solution will fill the syringe.

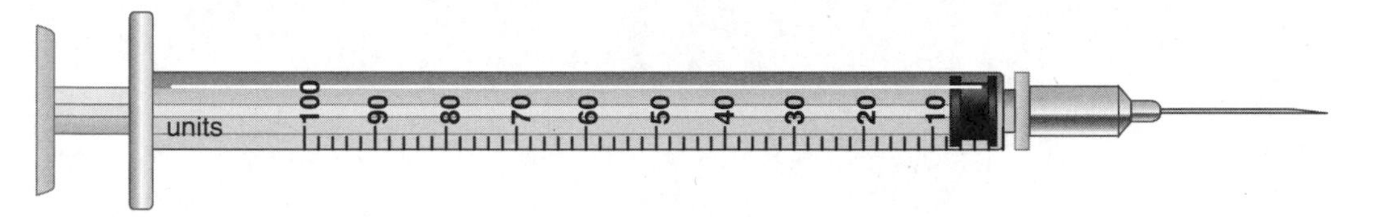

IMPLEMENT THE RACE MODEL: A CRITICAL-THINKING STRATEGY

Recognize keywords.	A patient has a prescription for **20 units** of NPH insulin and **6 units** of regular insulin to be administered subcutaneously at 0800. **Insert an arrow** at the line on the **barrel of the syringe** where the **total insulin solution will fill the syringe**.
Ask what the question is asking.	What is the total amount of units of insulin to be administered and where is this amount of solution on an insulin syringe?
Critically analyze each option in relation to the question and to the other options.	There are no options to consider in a Hot Spot item. The words in the stem that indicate that this is a hot spot question are *Insert an arrow*. To answer this question you must add the two doses of insulin (20 units + 6 units = 26 units) and then identify where the resulting single dose will be on an insulin syringe. **Rationales: The prescription is for 20 units of NPH insulin and 6 units of regular insulin. These medications can be combined into one syringe. The total dose is 26 units (20 units of NPH insulin and 6 units of regular insulin). Each line on this insulin syringe represents 2 units of insulin. Therefore, the answer should indicate that the total solution of insulin will reach line 26 on the insulin syringe.** units 100 90 80 70 60 50 40 30 20 10
Eliminate incorrect options.	There are no incorrect options presented.

SUMMARY

Thinking about thinking is more strenuous than physical labor. A physical task is always easier if you use the right tool. This concept also is true for mental labor. A critical-thinking strategy, such as the RACE model, provides a methodical, analytical approach to answering questions in nursing. As with any strategy, it takes practice and experience to perfect its use. Therefore, you are encouraged to use this critical-thinking strategy when practicing test taking or reviewing examinations.

2 Nursing Within the Context of Contemporary Health Care

Theory-Based Nursing Care

KEYWORDS

The following words include nursing/medical terminology, concepts, principles, and information relevant to content specifically addressed in the chapter or associated with topics presented in it. English dictionaries, nursing textbooks, and medical dictionaries, such as *Taber's Cyclopedic Medical Dictionary,* are resources that can be used to expand your knowledge and understanding of these words and related information.

Actualization
Adaptive capacity
Beliefs
Critical time
Defense mechanism
Developmental task
Erikson, Erik—Personality Development
Freud, Sigmund—Psychoanalytic Theory
Gordon, Marjorie—Functional Health Patterns
Health
Health belief
Health-illness continuum
Homeostasis
Human behavior
Jung, Carl—Personality Theory
Kübler-Ross, Elisabeth—Stages of Grieving
Libido
Maslow, Abraham—Hierarchy of Basic Human Needs
Model
Moral development
Multiplicity of stressors
Philosophy of nursing
Piaget, Jean—Theory of Cognitive Development
Stress
Stressor (primary, secondary)
Theory
Values
Wellness

THEORY-BASED NURSING CARE: QUESTIONS

1. A nurse is considering the Faith Development Theory by James Fowler while assessing several patients. Which patients does the nurse expect to assume responsibility for their own beliefs about faith?
1. Older adolescents
2. Young adolescents
3. Older school-age children
4. Young school-age children

2. A nurse is caring for a group of patients. A patient experiencing which of the following situations does the nurse anticipate will have the hardest time coping?
1. Scheduled for a biopsy
2. Unable to control the course of illness
3. Challenged by a multiplicity of stressors
4. Having to relocate to an assisted-living facility

3. A nurse inadvertently commits a medication error without the knowledge of other nursing team members. According to Freud, which part of the personality guides the nurse to initiate an Incident Report?
   1. Id
   2. Ego
   3. Libido
   4. Superego

4. Which statement does the nurse understand is related to adaptations associated with the General Adaptation Syndrome?
   1. Adaptations depend on the nature of the stressor.
   2. Adaptations can be conscious or unconscious.
   3. Adaptations become secondary stressors.
   4. Adaptations are maladaptive responses.

5. A patient with terminal cancer is willing to try new therapies. Which stage of Kübler-Ross Stages of Grieving does the nurse identify that the patient is experiencing?
   1. Denial
   2. Depression
   3. Bargaining
   4. Acceptance

6. A nurse gives a resident in a nursing home a choice about which color shirt to wear. Which level need, according to Maslow's Hierarchy of Needs, has the nurse just met?
   1. Self-esteem
   2. Physiological
   3. Safety and Security
   4. Love and Belonging

7. A nurse is assessing a child in relation to the stages of Jean Piaget's Theory of Cognitive Development. Which behavior indicates that the child has reached the Formal Operations stage of cognitive development according to Piaget?
   1. Employs logical thought to organize collected information
   2. Utilizes deductive reasoning to examine alternatives
   3. Explores objects by placing them in the mouth
   4. Uses language to communicate with others

8. Which statement **best** reflects a principle common to all theories of health, wellness, and illness?
   1. Health is synonymous with a sense of well-being.
   2. People are able to control factors that affect health.
   3. Many variables influence a person's perception of health.
   4. Being able to meet the demands of one's role is necessary for health.

9. According to Maslow, which characteristic is **least** associated with a person who is self-actualized?
   1. Is autonomous
   2. Is able to see the good in others
   3. Has the ability to problem-solve
   4. Has an external locus of control

10. Which concept identified by the nurse is basic to the health-illness continuum model?
    1. People can be both healthy and ill at the same time on the continuum.
    2. Actualization must be achieved to be on the healthy end of the continuum.
    3. When variables are balanced people are in the exact center of the continuum.
    4. There is no distinct boundary between health and illness along the continuum.

11. A prospective nurse is being interviewed for a job by the nurse manager in an urgent care center. The nurse manager states that the facility adheres to a clinical model of health/illness. Which should the nurse anticipate will be expected of the nurses within this facility?
   1. Consider patients as holistic human beings.
   2. Make assessment of patients in the physiological domain.
   3. Identify the relationship between patients' beliefs and actions.
   4. Recognize if patients are able to perform their role within the family.

12. Which person is considered healthy when referring to the Role-Performance Model of Health?
   1. Coal miner who retires after acquiring black lung disease
   2. Coach who continues to coach after becoming a paraplegic
   3. Brick layer who takes a leave of absence while recovering from hernia surgery
   4. Police officer who sells alarm systems after leaving the force because of being shot while on duty

13. Freedom from which situation demonstrates a safety and security need in Maslow's Hierarchy of Human Needs?
   1. Pain
   2. Hunger
   3. Ridicule
   4. Loneliness

14. A nurse is caring for patients who have experienced a variety of stressful life events. Which event has the greatest potential to contribute to stress-related illness?
   1. Retirement
   2. Pregnancy
   3. Adoption
   4. Divorce

15. A nurse is facilitating a support group for people who are coping with the death of a significant other. Which patient behavior reflects complicated grieving?
   1. Remarrying within 6 months after the death of a wife
   2. Being continuously angry 3 months after the death of a parent
   3. Keeping a child's room unchanged for 4 years after the death of the child
   4. Displaying clinical symptoms of depression 9 months after the death of a husband

16. A nurse identifies that love and belonging needs associated with Maslow's Hierarchy of Needs are related to which of Gordon's Functional Health Patterns?
   1. Values-belief pattern
   2. Role-relationship pattern
   3. Cognitive-perceptual pattern
   4. Sexuality-reproductive pattern

17. Which statement identifies a basic principle associated with Sigmund Freud and his work?
   1. The reality principle reflects man's need for immediate gratification.
   2. Defense mechanisms are a common means of conscious coping.
   3. The id controls the personality.
   4. No behavior is accidental.

18. Which concept about health do nurses need to appreciate?
   1. Perceptions of health vary among cultures.
   2. To be considered healthy a person needs to be productive.
   3. There must be an absence of illness for a person to be considered healthy.
   4. Underlying consensus exists among theorists about the definition of health.

19. A nurse is caring for an immobilized patient who was admitted to the hospital with a pressure ulcer. Which type of stressor precipitated the pressure ulcer?
1. Microbiological
2. Physiological
3. Chemical
4. Physical

20. The Health Belief Model attempts to explain and predict health behaviors and focuses on which of the following?
1. One's ability to fulfill one's assigned roles
2. Constructs associated with perceived threat and net benefit
3. Locus of control being important in one making choices about health behaviors
4. People moving along a continuum from health on one end to illness on the other end

21. A nurse is assessing a patient who is experiencing prolonged stress. For which **most** serious complication should the nurse monitor the patient?
1. Altered sleeping
2. Impaired immunity
3. Increased muscle tension
4. Decreased intestinal peristalsis

22. A nurse is analyzing information about a patient. Which of the following does Maslow's Hierarchy of Needs theory help the nurse to identify?
1. Patient's problem that has top priority
2. Developmental level of the patient
3. Coping patterns of the patient
4. Patient's health beliefs

23. A nurse is teaching a course about death and dying to a community group. Which is **most** important for the nurse to teach parents about preparing a child for the death of a grandparent?
1. Wait until the child asks a question about the situation.
2. Encourage the child to participate in mourning rituals.
3. Begin at the child's level of understanding.
4. Praise the child for being strong.

24. A nurse is assessing a patient who experienced an emotional stress. Which **most** common response should the nurse anticipate the patient will exhibit?
1. Anger
2. Denial
3. Anxiety
4. Depression

25. A nurse is assessing patients in the postanesthesia care unit. For which physiological responses to stress should the nurse monitor this patient? **Select all that apply.**
1. _____Dilated pupils
2. _____Slow, bounding pulse
3. _____Delayed response time
4. _____Inability to concentrate
5. _____Rapid, shallow breathing
6. _____Increased muscle tension

26. Which nursing interventions support a problem in the Role-Relationship Pattern category of Gordon's Functional Health Patterns? **Select all that apply.**
1. _____Seeking the assistance of a spiritual advisor
2. _____Teaching the patient self-care in preparation for going home
3. _____Referring a patient to a self-help group to learn colostomy care
4. _____Assessing a family member's readiness to provide care in the home
5. _____Protecting a patient from family members who disagree with the patient's medical choices

27. A nurse is differentiating between primary and secondary stressors. Which stressors are examples of secondary stressors? **Select all that apply.**
1. _____Pain
2. _____Cold weather
3. _____Death of a spouse
4. _____Shortness of breath
5. _____Ingested microorganisms
6. _____Increased blood pressure

28. Of the patients presented, which patient's level of wellness does the nurse determine best represents the placement of the X on Dunn's Health Grid?

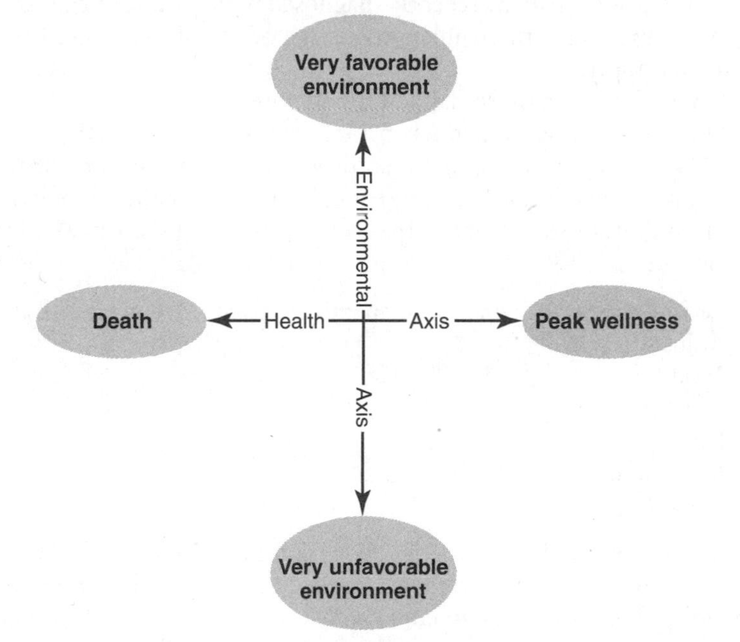

1. A healthy, active older adult who has an apartment in an independent living facility that provides daily meals, weekly housekeeping, and services such as activities, medical and dental care on site, and banking available 2 days a week
2. A person with a diagnosis of diabetes with a stable blood glucose who receives weekly visits from a public health nurse and has a home health aide who visits three mornings a week
3. A person with a diagnosis of stage II-A lung cancer who lives in a men's shelter and who consistently misses clinic appointments
4. A relatively healthy homeless person with a diagnosis of pneumonia and who is responding to medication

29. Which are examples of a health belief? **Select all that apply.**
1. _____Eating foods that are low in fat
2. _____Accepting grim results of diagnostic tests
3. _____Concluding that illness is the result of being bad
4. _____Recognizing that smoking can cause lung cancer
5. _____Respecting a patient's decision regarding therapeutic treatment

30. Which are examples of a response to a physiological stressor? **Select all that apply.**
1. _____A sunburn after being outside all day
2. _____Diarrhea after eating contaminated food
3. _____Shortness of breath when walking up a hill
4. _____A rapid heart rate during a final examination
5. _____Fluid volume excess as a result of renal disease

31. The Kübler-Ross Stages of Grieving theory reflects a process that progresses through several stages to final acceptance. List these patient statements in order according to the Kübler-Ross Stages of Grieving.
1. "I am going to get a second opinion."
2. "I find it so hard to think about the fact that I don't have long to live."
3. "I've never smoked in my life. I shouldn't be the one with lung cancer."
4. "I'll have the chemotherapy because I want to see my children grow up."
5. "I don't want a big funeral because I want people to remember me and be happy."

Answer: ____________________

32. A nurse is caring for a patient recently diagnosed with advanced cancer. Which patient statements reflect the Kübler-Ross stage of denial in the grief process? **Select all that apply.**
1. _____"Why did this have to happen to me now?"
2. _____"How could this happen when I quit smoking cigarettes?"
3. _____"Maybe they mixed up my records with someone else's records."
4. _____"I probably will not live long enough to see my children married."
5. _____"I don't want to talk about the fact that they tell me I have advanced cancer."

33. Which words describe the concept of adaptive capacity? **Select all that apply.**
1. _____Adjust
2. _____Modify
3. _____Change
4. _____Etiology
5. _____Remission
6. _____Compliance

34. A nurse educator is conducting a class about child development for nurses. The nurse reviews the Stages of Moral Development Theory by Lawrence Kohlberg. Place the following patient statements about what motivates them to behave that reflects the reasoning typical of progression through Kohlberg's stages of moral development.
1. "I was following the rules."
2. "I did not want to get punished."
3. "I expected to receive a reward."
4. "I thought it was the right thing to do."
5. "I wanted others to see me as a good person."
6. "I was doing what is acceptable in our community."

Answer: ____________________

35. A nurse is caring for a newly admitted patient. The nurse collects data and reviews the patient's clinical record. Which level need is the priority for this patient according to Maslow's Hierarchy of Needs?
1. Physiologic
2. Self-esteem
3. Safety and security
4. Love and belonging

PATIENT'S CLINICAL RECORD

Vital Signs

Temperature: 99.8°F, temporal
Pulse: 110 beats per minute
Respirations: 24 breaths per minute

Pain Assessment

Reports a pain level of 9 on a scale of 0 to 10
"Sharp, piercing pain"
Located in lower left abdomen
Pain started 3 days ago and became progressively worse

Social History

Sixty-five-year-old female
Smokes 1 pack of cigarettes daily for 45 years
Drinks alcohol socially on weekends
Husband of 45 years died of colon cancer 1 year ago
States that she "misses him a lot"
Daughter wants her to move in with her but patient states she wants to remain independent because she is able to take care of herself
Participates in a sewing group at her church making pillowcases for hospitalized children

THEORY-BASED NURSING CARE: ANSWERS AND RATIONALES

1. 1. **Older adolescents and young adults assume responsibility for their own commitments, beliefs, and attitudes about faith. This reflects the individuative-reflective stage of faith development.**
   2. Young adolescents begin to examine life-guiding beliefs, values, and attitudes about faith. This reflects the synthetic-conventional stage of faith development.
   3. Older school-age children may accept the concept of God and appreciate the perceptions of others. This reflects the mythic-literal stage of faith development.
   4. Children between 3 and 7 years of age imitate parental behaviors without thorough understanding. This reflects the intuitive-projective stage of faith development.

2. 1. Although waiting for the results of a biopsy is stressful, it is not as stressful as one of the other options offered.
   2. Although being unable to control the course of illness is stressful, it is not as stressful as one of the other options offered.
   3. **As the multiplicity of stressors increases, it becomes harder for a person to cope. As each stress is added, the accumulated impact is greater than just the sum of each individual stressor.**
   4. Relocation is stressful whether it is voluntary or involuntary. However, it is not as stressful as one of the other options offered.

3. 1. The id will not guide a nurse to initiate an incident report because the id is the source of instinctive and unconscious urges, not the center of the conscience.
   2. The ego seeks compromise between the id and superego and represents the psychological aspect of the personality, not the center of the conscience.
   3. Libido refers to the psychic energy derived from basic biological urges, not the center of the conscience.
   4. **The superego monitors the ego. The superego is concerned with social standards, ethics, self-criticism, moral standards, and conscience. If the nurse initiates an Incident Report, it is the superego that directs the achievement of ego-ideal behavior. If the nurse does not initiate an Incident Report, it is the superego that criticizes, punishes, and causes a sense of guilt.**

4. 1. The General and Local Adaptation Syndromes involve automatic nonspecific responses that are not dependent on specific stressors. The body automatically responds in the same way physiologically regardless of the nature of the stressor.
   2. **Reactions to stress are both conscious and unconscious. In the General and Local Adaptation Syndromes, automatic physiological responses are not under conscious control. Adaptations, such as behavioral responses, are often under conscious control.**
   3. Although an adaptation may become a secondary stressor, many do not.
   4. Adaptations can be maladaptive and fail to help a person achieve or maintain balance or they can be positive and help a person achieve or maintain balance.

5. 1. A patient in the denial stage of grieving refuses to believe that the event is happening and is unable to deal with practical problems such as trying new therapies.
   2. A patient in the depression stage of grieving usually will acknowledge the reality and inevitability of the impending loss, will grieve the loss of present relationships and future experiences, and may stop all but palliative therapy.
   3. **A patient in the bargaining stage of grieving seeks to avoid the loss and will try new therapies to gain more time.**
   4. A patient in the acceptance stage of grieving comes to terms with the loss. The patient begins to detach from surroundings and supportive people and generally no longer has the emotional or physical energy to try new therapies.

6. 1. **Choosing which color shirt to wear provides a person with the opportunity to make a choice and supports feelings of independence, competence, and self-respect, which all contribute to a positive self-esteem.**

2. Providing choices does not meet needs on the physiological level of Maslow's Hierarchy of Needs. Physiological needs are related to having adequate air, food, water, rest, shelter, and the ability to eliminate and regulate body temperature.
3. Providing choices does not meet needs on the safety and security level of Maslow's Hierarchy of Needs. Safety and security needs are related to being and feeling protected in the physiological and interpersonal realms.
4. Providing choices does not meet needs on the love and belonging level of Maslow's Hierarchy of Needs. Love and belonging needs are related to giving and receiving affection, attempting to avoid loneliness and isolation, and wanting to feel as though one belongs.

7. 1. Employing logical thought to organize information reflects the Concrete Operations stage of cognitive development. These individuals use logical thought to organize information and solve concrete problems. Also, they are less egocentric than when in previous stages.
2. Using deductive reasoning to examine alternatives reflects the Formal Operations stage of cognitive development. These individuals use symbols related to abstract concepts and are capable of hypothetical and deductive reasoning.
3. Exploring objects by placing them in the mouth reflects the Sensorimotor stage of cognitive development. These individuals process information on the physical or emotional level primarily through the senses.
4. Using language to communicate with others reflects the Preoperational stage of cognitive development. These individuals demonstrate an increasing ability to connect cognitively through language and actions.

8. 1. Not all models of health agree with this view of health. For example, the Clinical Model has a narrow interpretation that views health as the absence of signs and symptoms of disease or injury. Well-being is a subjective perception of energy and vigor. A person able to carry out daily tasks, interact successfully with others, manage stress and emotions, and strive for continued growth and who has meaning or purpose in life has a sense of well-being, regardless of the severity of disease or infirmity.
2. Not all definitions of health identify that a person is able to control factors that affect health. The Adaptive Model is one of the few that addresses a person's ability to use purposeful adaptive responses and processes in response to internal and external stimuli to achieve health.
3. There is little consensus about any one definition of health, wellness, and illness. However, all definitions of health, wellness, and illness address the fact that there are a number of factors that influence health.
4. Not all definitions of health define health in terms of an individual's ability to fulfill societal roles. For example, the Clinical Model views people from the perspective of a physiological system with related functions with health being the absence of disease or injury.

9. 1. Self-actualized people are autonomous, independent, self-directed, and governed from within.
2. Self-actualized people are friendly and loving. They respect themselves and others and seek out the good in others.
3. Self-actualized people are accurate in predicting future events, highly creative, and open to new ideas and have superior perception. All these qualities contribute to problem-solving abilities.
4. An external locus of control least describes self-actualized people. People with an external locus of control respond to a reward or recognition that comes from outside the self. People who are self-actualized strive to develop their maximum potential based on motivation from within.

10. 1. Where people place themselves on the health-illness continuum is a self-perception of their status in relation to health and illness. From their perspectives they cannot be healthy and ill at the same time.
2. Only the Eudaemonistic Model of Health incorporates the concept of actualization or realization of a person's potential as the major component of a definition of health.

3. Variables, such as genetic makeup, race, gender, age, lifestyle, risk factors, culture, environment, standard of living, support system, spiritual beliefs, and emotional factors, may be in balance and individuals may view themselves at the extremes of the continuum or they may be out of balance and view themselves in the center of the continuum.
4. **Health and illness are on opposite ends of the health-illness continuum and there is no distinct boundary between health and illness. Only a person can place herself or himself somewhere along the health-illness continuum based on his or her own perceptions about what constitutes health and illness.**

11. 1. Holistic health care involves viewing all dimensions of the person including emotional, mental, spiritual, and physical. This is a broad approach when compared with the clinical model.
2. **The clinical model, also known as the medical model, is concerned with the presence or absence of signs and symptoms of illness, disease, or injury. It is a narrow interpretation of health/illness because the focus is on the identification and treatment of a defect or dysfunction. Urgent care centers are concerned with meeting acute health-care needs.**
3. Identifying the relationship between patients' beliefs and actions is a component of the Health Belief Model of Health Behavior. It is unrelated to the clinical model of health/illness.
4. Performing societal roles (e.g., parent, spouse, friend, and employee) is related to the Role Performance Model of Health. It is a narrow interpretation of health and is unrelated to the clinical model of health/illness.

12. 1. If a person retires because of illness, the person has not met society's expectation in terms of role performance and, therefore, is considered unhealthy in light of the Role-Performance Model of Health.
2. **According to the Role-Performance Model of Health, as long as a person can perform work associated with societal roles, even if a person is limited physically, the person is considered healthy. A coach who continues coaching even though ill or disabled is considered healthy in light of the Role-Performance Model of Health.**
3. According to the Role-Performance Model of Health, a person who cannot fulfill responsibilities associated with one's job is considered sick. Therefore, a person who takes a leave of absence from work to recover is someone who is considered unhealthy in this model.
4. A strict interpretation of the Role-Performance Model of Health will most likely describe a police officer who changes jobs because of a physical or emotional inability to continue the first job as unhealthy. Even though the former police officer is still a wage earner, it is not in the same job.

13. 1. **According to Maslow's Hierarchy of Needs, freedom from pain is considered a safety and security need. Confusion sometimes occurs because other theorists, such as R. A. Kalish, believe that pain should be categorized along with adequate air, food, water, rest/sleep, shelter, elimination, and temperature regulation as a first-level physiological need.**
2. According to Maslow's Hierarchy of Needs, freedom from hunger is considered a first-level physiological need, not a safety and security need.
3. According to Maslow's Hierarchy of Needs, freedom from ridicule is associated with self-esteem needs, not safety and security needs.
4. According to Maslow's Hierarchy of Needs, freedom from loneliness is associated with the need to feel loved and to belong, not to feel safe and secure.

14. 1. According to the Social Readjustment Rating Scale by Holmes and Rahe, retirement is ranked 10th on the list of life events likely to cause stress-related illness with a life-change unit score of 45 of 100. Retirement is considered less stressful than one of the other options offered.
2. According to the Social Readjustment Rating Scale by Holmes and Rahe, pregnancy is ranked 12th on the list of life events likely to cause stress-related illness with a life-change unit score of 40 of 100. Pregnancy is considered less stressful than two other options offered.

3. According to the Social Readjustment Rating Scale by Holmes and Rahe, the gaining of a new family member is ranked 14th on the list of life events likely to cause stress-related illness with a life-change unit score of 39 of 100. All of the other options are considered more stressful than gaining a new family member.
4. **According to the Social Readjustment Rating Scale by Holmes and Rahe, divorce is ranked second on the list of life events likely to cause stress-related illness with a life-change unit score of 73 of 100. Only death of a spouse, ranked first on the scale with a score of 100, is considered more stressful than divorce.**

15. 1. Moving on with one's life is a sign of successful grieving. Mourning periods may be abbreviated if the loss is replaced immediately by another equally respected person or if the person experienced anticipatory grieving, which is grieving experienced before the death.
2. Being continuously angry 3 months after the death of a parent is within the realm of expected grieving behavior and is not complicated grieving. If a person is continuously angry after 1 year, it is considered complicated grieving.
3. **Keeping a deceased child's room unchanged for years is outside the usual limits of grieving. Often a person can get stuck in a stage of grieving and is unable to progress to the next stage. Keeping a room unchanged for years reflects an inability to face the reality of the loss or to deal with the feelings associated with the loss.**
4. Depression of this length is not uncommon, particularly if the relationship was meaningful or intense or no one was able to fill the role of the deceased. If depression does not resolve within a year after the death, it is considered complicated grieving.

16. 1. Love and belonging needs identified in Maslow's Hierarchy of Needs are not associated with Gordon's Value-Belief Pattern category. Gordon's Value-Belief Pattern category addresses topics such as spiritual distress and well-being, not love and belonging needs.
2. **Love and belonging needs identified in Maslow's Hierarchy of Needs are associated with Gordon's Role-Relationship Pattern category. Gordon's Role-Relationship Pattern category addresses topics such as social issues, loneliness, and relationships among family members and others.**
3. Love and belonging needs identified in Maslow's Hierarchy of Needs are not associated with Gordon's Cognitive-Perceptual Pattern category. Gordon's Cognitive-Perceptual Pattern category addresses topics such as comfort, confusion, conflict, knowledge deficit, disturbed thought processes, and sensory perception, not love and belonging needs.
4. Love and belonging needs identified in Maslow's Hierarchy of Needs are not associated with Gordon's Sexuality-Reproduction Pattern category. Gordon's Sexuality-Reproduction Pattern category addresses topics such as altered sexuality patterns and dysfunction, not love and belonging needs.

17. 1. The reality principle according to Freud is a learned ego function whereby a person is able to delay the need for pleasure rather than seek immediate gratification.
2. Defense mechanisms are unconscious, not conscious, coping patterns that deny, distort, or reduce awareness of a stressful event in an attempt to protect the personality from anxiety.
3. The ego, not the id, controls the personality. The ego mediates the urges of the id and the conscience of the superego and is therefore the part of the psyche that controls the personality.
4. **Freud believed that all behavior has meaning and called this theory psychic determinism. He believed that every psychic event is determined by prior events. Behavior, mental phenomena, and even dreams are not accidental but rather an expression of thoughts, feelings, or needs that have a relationship to the rest of a person's life.**

18. **1. Every individual is influenced by family, ethnic, and cultural beliefs and values. These beliefs and values influence a person's lifestyle through how one perceives, experiences, and copes with health, illness, and disability. The nurse must assess the impact of these influences on the patient's health and health practices.**

2. Only in the Role-Performance Model of Health is productivity or performance of one's role a necessary component to be considered healthy. While important to understand, it is a narrow definition of health and fails to include the multitude of other factors that impact on a definition of health.
3. Absence of disease or injury is the foundation of the Clinical Model of Health and fails to include the multitude of other factors that impact on a definition of health.
4. Health cannot be easily measured or defined in common terms. There is no consensus on a definition of health, because health is unique to each individual and is based on personal expectations and values.

19. 1. Pressure is not a microbiological stressor. Microbiological stressors precipitate infection.
2. Pressure is not a physiological stressor. Physiological stressors are disturbances in structure or function of any tissue, organ, system, or body part.
3. Pressure is not a chemical stressor. Chemical stressors are drugs, poisons, and toxins.
4. The force of pressure is a physical stressor. Pressure is the continuous force of a body part on a surface as a result of gravity; compression of tissue occurs between a bony prominence and the surface on which the body part is resting. This force is external to the body. The pressure ulcer, which is the response, becomes a secondary stressor that is then physiological in nature.

20. 1. Fulfilling one's roles is the focus of the Role-Performance Model of Health and Wellness. This model states that health is defined in terms of a person's ability to fulfill societal roles; if roles are met, people perceive themselves as healthy even if they have an illness.
2. The Health Belief Model focuses on perceived threats, severity, benefits, barriers, cues to action, and self-efficacy, which all influence a person's "readiness to act" in response to a health threat; Rosenstock first proposed this model during the 1950s.
3. Locus of control is the focus of the Health Locus of Control Model. If the nurse knows that a patient is motivated by either internal or external forces, then the nurse can plan internal or external reinforcement training to motivate a patient toward better health.
4. This is the focus of the health-illness continuum Model of Health and Wellness. This model focuses on health being on one end of the continuum and illness being on the other end. People move back and forth along the continuum based on their own perceptions with no distinct boundary between health and illness.

21. 1. Difficulty sleeping is a common response to stress, but it is not life-threatening. Although it can contribute to fatigue, it is not as serious a concern as one of the other options offered.
2. Impaired immunity is a serious threat caused by prolonged periods of stress. Stressors elevate blood cortisone levels, which decrease anti-inflammatory responses, deplete energy stores, lead to a state of exhaustion, and decrease resistance to disease.
3. Increased muscle tension is a physiological indicator of stress. However, it is not as serious a concern as one of the other options offered.
4. When stressed, the patient's parasympathetic nervous system precipitates a decrease in intestinal peristalsis. Constipation is a concern, but it is not as serious as one of the other options offered.

22. 1. Patient problems/needs can be ranked in order of ascending importance according to how essential they are for survival using Maslow's Hierarchy of Needs as a framework. Maslow identifies five levels of human needs. A person must meet lower-level needs before addressing higher-level needs. Physiological needs are first-level needs: air, food, water, sleep, shelter, etc.; safety and security needs are second; love and belonging needs are third; self-esteem needs are fourth; and self-actualization is the fifth-level need.
2. Erikson's Developmental Theory is designed to identify a patient's developmental level, not Maslow's Hierarchy of Needs.
3. Maslow's Hierarchy of Needs is not designed to identify a person's coping patterns in response to illness.

4. Rosenstock's and Becker's Health Belief Models, not Maslow's Hierarchy of Needs, identify the relationship between health beliefs and the use of preventive actions to promote health.

23. 1. Waiting until the child asks a question is not an effective way to deal with childhood grieving. Children are perceptive and capable of recognizing that something is wrong but may not know what questions to ask. Avoiding discussing the loss with the child, may make the child feel afraid, lonely, or even abandoned.
2. The child's age, level of understanding, feelings, and fears will determine how much the child should engage in mourning rituals. Children should not be forced to attend mourning rituals, nor should they be pushed aside in an attempt to protect them from pain, because this can lead to feelings of abandonment, fear, or loneliness.
3. Beginning at the child's level of understanding is essential when preparing a child for the death of a grandparent. Because there is such a difference regarding how children of different ages view the concept of death, it is important first to assess the child's level of understanding.
4. No one should be told how to feel or behave when it comes to reacting to loss. Expression of diverse feelings is essential if a child is to cope with the loss of the grandparent or develop positive coping strategies to deal with loss later as an adult.

24. 1. Although anger may be identified as a reaction to stress, it is not the most common response to stress. Anger is more classically seen in the Kübler-Ross second stage of dying/grieving.
2. Denial is more commonly seen in the Kübler-Ross first stage of dying/grieving, not as the most common response to stress.
3. Anxiety is the most common response to all new experiences that serve as an emotional threat.
4. Depression is an extreme response to prolonged stress and is not the most common human response to stress.

25. 1. Dilated pupils increase visual perception in reaction to a perceived threat.
2. Whereas a bounding pulse is a physiological response to stress, a rapid pulse, not a slow pulse, is a physiological response to the body's neurohormonal reaction to stress. During the alarm phase of the General Adaptation Syndrome, the autonomic nervous system initiates the fight-or-flight response and releases large amounts of epinephrine and cortisone into the body that contribute to a rapid pulse.
3. The response time is shorter, not longer, when a person is exposed to a stressor as a result of an increase in alertness and energy associated with the alarm phase of the General Adaptation syndrome. In addition, level of alertness is considered a psychosocial, not physiological, response to stress.
4. Concentration is considered a psychosocial, not physiological, response to stress. Concentration and level of alertness are enhanced, not reduced, during the fight-or-flight response of the autonomic nervous system when large amounts of epinephrine and cortisone are released into the body.
5. Rapid, shallow breathing is a physiological response associated with the fight-or-flight response of the autonomic nervous system when large amounts of cortisone and epinephrine are released into the body as a person perceives a threat.
6. Increased muscle tension prepares the body for fight or flight.

26. 1. This action supports the achievement of a goal in the Value-Belief category, not the Role-Relationship category.
2. This action supports achievement of a goal in the Cognitive-Perceptual category, not the Role-Relationship category.
3. This action supports the achievement of a goal in the Health Perception/Health Management category, not the Role-Relationship category.
4. This action supports achievement of a goal in the Role-Relationship category.
5. This action supports achievement of a goal in the Role-Relationship category. Patients have a right to make medical decisions for themselves.

27. 1. Pain initially is a response to some previous primary stressor, threat, or

stimuli. However, when pain stimulates additional responses in an effort to manage the pain, the pain becomes a secondary stressor.

2. Cold weather is a primary physical stressor, not a response to some previous stressor.
3. Death of a spouse is a primary psychosocial stressor, not a response to some previous stressor.
4. **Shortness of breath is a response to a primary stressor such as cancer of the lung or a respiratory tract infection. Shortness of breath then becomes a secondary stressor precipitating further adaptations in the individual.**
5. Ingested microorganisms are a primary microbiological stressor, not a response to some previous stressor.
6. **Increased blood pressure is a secondary stressor. It is in response to a primary stressor such as a systemic infection or fear of the unknown.**

28. 1. This person is healthy, active, and lives in a favorable, supportive environment. This person reflects high-level wellness and should be plotted on the upper right side of Dunn's Health Grid.

2. **This person is in poor health but receives routine care from health team members. This person reflects protected poor health and should be plotted on the upper left side of Dunn's Health Grid.**

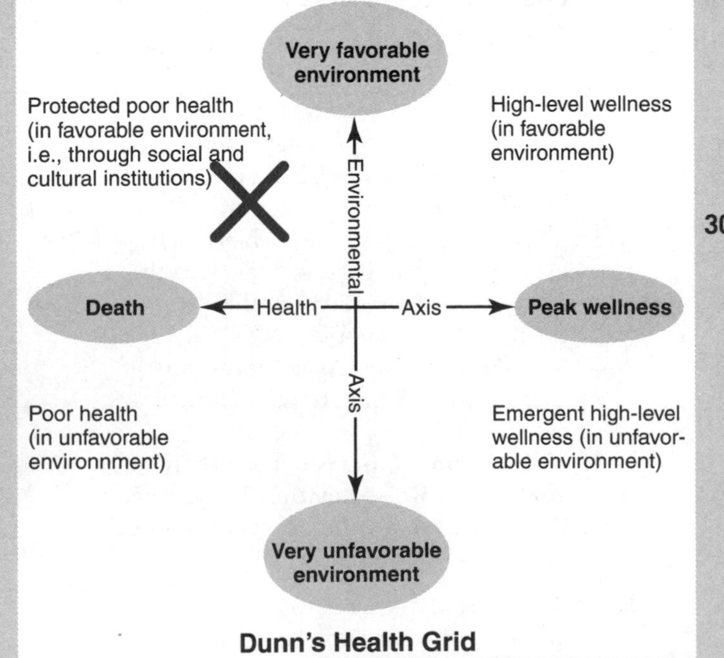

Dunn's Health Grid

3. This person has a chronic health problem, is not receiving consistent heath care, and lives in a men's shelter. This person reflects poor health and lives in an unfavorable environment and should be plotted on the lower left side of Dunn's Health Grid.
4. This person is relatively healthy and is recovering from pneumonia but is homeless, which is an environment that is unfavorable. This person reflects emergent high-level wellness and should be plotted on the lower right side of Dunn's Health Grid.

29. 1. Eating foods low in fat is a health practice, not a health belief. A health behavior, such as eating a low-fat diet, reflects the belief that preventive measures will minimize risk factors that contribute to disease/illness.

2. Accepting grim results of diagnostic tests reflects a behavior in response to bad news, rather than a behavior reflecting a health belief.
3. **This is an example of a health belief. A health belief is a conviction or opinion that influences health-care practices or decisions. If a person believes that illness is the result of being bad, the person may feel the need to suffer in silence as a form of penance.**
4. **This is an example of a health belief. If a person believes that smoking cigarettes can cause lung cancer, then the person may refrain from smoking.**
5. Respecting a patient's decision is not an example of a health belief. It reflects the nurse's acceptance of a patient as a unique individual and recognizes the patient's right to make personal choices about health care.

30. 1. A sunburn is a response to the ultraviolet rays of the sun, which is a physical, not a physiological, stressor. Once the person has a sunburn, the sunburn is a physiological stressor.

2. Diarrhea after eating contaminated food is a response to a microbiological, not a physiological, stressor.
3. **Shortness of breath is a response to the physiological stress of walking up a hill. The body is reacting via physiological mechanisms to take in more oxygen to meet the oxygen demand of cells when walking.**

4. The threat of a final examination is a psychological, not a physiological, stressor. The rapid heart rate during a final examination is a physiological response to a psychological stressor.
5. Fluid volume excess is a response to the physiological stress of kidney impairment. Because of impaired kidney function the body is unable to secrete urine and fluid, volume excess occurs.

31. 1. This statement reflects "doctor shopping," which is a form of denial, the first stage of the Kübler-Ross Stages of Grieving theory. The patient is experiencing shock and disbelief.
3. This statement reflects the anger stage, the second stage of the Kübler-Ross Stages of Grieving theory. The patient is aware of the reality of the situation and is resentful and angry.
4. This statement characterizes the bargaining stage, the third stage of the Kübler-Ross Stages of Grieving theory. The patient is negotiating for more time.
2. This statement reflects depression, the fourth stage of the Kübler-Ross Stages of Grieving theory. The patient is grieving over what is happening and what will never be.
5. This statement characterizes acceptance, the fifth stage of the Kübler-Ross Stages of Grieving theory. The patient has accepted the inevitable and is looking toward the future.

32. 1. This statement characterizes the anger, not denial, stage in the grieving process. During the anger stage the person may vent hostile feelings or displace these feelings on others through acting out behaviors.
2. This statement characterizes the anger, not denial, stage of the grieving process. During the anger stage the person may question, "Why me when I did everything right?"
3. This statement characterizes the denial stage of the grieving process. When in denial a patient may identify reasons why the diagnosis is not possible.
4. This statement characterizes the depression stage of the grieving process. During the depression stage the patient realizes the full impact of the situation and grieves future losses.
5. This statement characterizes the denial stage of the grieving process. The patient is using the defense mechanism of suppression. During denial the person is not ready to address or believe that the loss is happening.

33. 1. Adaptive capacity refers to the quality and quantity of resources one can draw on to regain balance after one is threatened. This process requires an individual to adjust consciously or unconsciously in the physical, emotional, mental, or spiritual dimension in an effort to achieve balance or homeostasis.
2. Adaptive capacity refers to the quality and quantity of resources one can draw on to regain balance after one is threatened. This process requires an individual to modify consciously or unconsciously in the physical, emotional, mental, or spiritual dimension in an effort to achieve balance or homeostasis.
3. Adaptive capacity refers to the quality and quantity of resources one can draw on to regain balance after one is threatened. This process requires an individual to change consciously or unconsciously in the physical, emotional, mental, or spiritual dimension in an effort to achieve balance or homeostasis.
4. Etiology refers to the stressor or threat to homeostasis that stimulates a person to draw on personal resources within the physical, emotional, mental, or spiritual dimension.
5. Remission refers to the abatement or lessened intensity of the symptoms of a disease or illness, not adaptive capacity.
6. Compliance refers to adherence to an established therapeutic action plan, not adaptive capacity.

34. 2. The first stage of moral development is Obedience and Punishment. The motivation for behavior is fear of negative consequences (e.g., punishment, disapproval).
3. The second stage of moral development is Individualism and Exchange. The motivation for behavior is the desire for a positive consequence (e.g., reward, good result).

5. **The third stage of moral development is Interpersonal Relationships. The motivation for behavior is based on pleasing others because it is what others expect.**
1. **The fourth stage of moral development is Maintaining Social Order. The motivation for behavior is based on following the rules to uphold the law.**
6. **The fifth stage of moral development is Social Contract and Individual Rights. The motivation for behavior is based on differing beliefs and values but adheres to standards agreed upon by society.**
4. **The sixth stage of moral development is Universal Principles. Motivation for behavior is based on abstract reasoning, universal ethical principles, and principles of justice.**

35. 1. A need in the *physiologic* level is not the priority. Although the pulse and respiratory rates are slightly higher than the expected (normal), ranges they are most likely a response to the pain experienced by the patient.
2. There are no data to support the conclusion that a need in the *self-esteem* level exists. The patient reports that she wants to remain independent and is able to care for herself.
3. **Pain is a *safety and security* level need based on Maslow's Hierarchy of Needs. Pain relief is the patient's priority need.**
4. A need in the *love and belonging* level is not the priority. The patient's daughter appears to be concerned about the patient's well-being. However the patient disagrees with moving in with her daughter.

Legal and Ethical Issues

KEYWORDS

The following words include nursing/medical terminology, concepts, principles, and information relevant to content specifically addressed in the chapter or associated with topics presented in it. English dictionaries, nursing textbooks, and medical dictionaries, such as *Taber's Cyclopedic Medical Dictionary,* are resources that can be used to expand your knowledge and understanding of these words and related information.

Accountability
Accreditation
Act of commission/omission
Advanced directives:
  Do Not Resuscitate
  Health-care proxy
  Power of attorney
American Nurses Association Standards of Nursing Practice
Assault
Battery
Beneficence
Breach of duty
Certification
Civil law
Code of Ethics
Common law
Confidentiality
Contract
Controlled substances
Crime
Criterion, Criteria
Defamation
Defendant
Defense
Ethics
Euthanasia
False imprisonment
Fraud
Functions of the nurse:
  Dependent
  Independent
  Interdependent
Good Samaritan law
Health-Care Quality Improvement Act
Incident Report
Informed consent
Invasion of privacy
Liability
Libel
Licensure
Litigation
Malpractice
National Council Licensing Examinations (NCLEX)
National League for Nursing Accrediting Commission
Negligence
Nonmaleficence
Nurse Practice Act
Occupational Safety and Health Acts (OSHA)
Patient Care Partnership (formerly called Patient's Bill of Rights)
Plaintiff
Professional liability insurance
Quality of life
Reciprocity
Res ipsa loquitur
Respondeat superior
Risk management
Sigma Theta Tau International, Honor Society of Nursing
Slander
Standards of care
State Board of Nursing
The Joint Commission (formerly the Joint Commission on Accreditation of Healthcare Organizations)
Tort
Veracity

LEGAL AND ETHICAL ISSUES: QUESTIONS

1. When a nurse is administering a medication to a confused patient, the patient says, "This pill looks different from the one I had before." Which should the nurse do?
1. Ask what the other pill looked like.
2. Explain the purpose of the medication.
3. Check the original medication prescription.
4. Encourage the patient to take the medication.

2. A nurse administers an incorrect dose of a medication to a patient. Which is the primary purpose of documenting this event in an Incident Report?
1. Record the event for future litigation.
2. Provide a basis for designing new policies.
3. Prevent similar situations from happening again.
4. Ensure accountability for the cause of the accident.

3. When preparing to administer a medication the nurse identifies that the dose is larger than the standard dose recommended by the manufacturer. Which should the nurse do?
1. Inform the supervisor.
2. Give the drug as prescribed.
3. Give the average dose of the medication.
4. Discuss the prescription with the primary health-care provider.

4. When a nurse attempts to administer a medication to a patient, the patient refuses to take the medication because it causes diarrhea. The nurse provides teaching about the medication, but the patient continues adamantly to refuse the medication. Which should the nurse do **first**?
1. Document the patient's refusal to take the medication.
2. Discuss with a family member the need for the patient to take the medication.
3. Explain again to the patient the consequences of refusing to take the medication.
4. Notify the primary health-care provider of the patient's refusal to take the medication.

5. When caring for a terminally ill patient a family member says, "I need your help to hasten my mother's death so that she is no longer suffering." Which should the nurse do, based on the position of the American Nurses Association in relation to assisted suicide?
1. Not participate in active euthanasia
2. Participate based on personal values and beliefs
3. Participate when the patient is experiencing severe pain
4. Not participate unless two primary health-care providers are consulted and the patient has had counseling

6. Which organization is responsible for ensuring that Registered Nurses are minimally qualified to practice nursing?
1. State Boards of Nursing
2. American Nurses Association
3. Sigma Theta Tau International
4. Constituent Leagues of the National League for Nursing

7. For which primary reason is a nurse expert called to testify in a lawsuit regarding professional nursing malpractice?
1. Strengthen the defense
2. Support the prosecution
3. Present standards of nursing care as they apply to the facts in the case
4. Make judgments associated with laws governing the practice of nursing

8. A nurse initiates a visit from a member of the clergy for a patient. How is the nurse functioning when initiating this visit?
1. Interdependently
2. Independently
3. Dependently
4. Collegially

9. A patient is asked to participate in a medical research study. Which document should the nurse explain to the patient because it protects the patient's rights?
1. Code of Ethics
2. Informed Consent
3. Nurse Practice Act
4. Constitution of the United States

10. Which element of ethical practice is associated with fair policies and procedures guiding allocation of organs for transplantation?
1. Justice
2. Fidelity
3. Veracity
4. Nonmaleficence

11. A primary health-care provider orders out of bed to a chair as the activity level for a patient. How is the nurse functioning when moving this patient out of bed to a chair?
1. Interdependently
2. Collaboratively
3. Independently
4. Dependently

12. A Registered Nurse witnesses an accident and assists the victim who has a life-threatening injury. Which should the nurse do to meet an important standard of care when acting as a Good Samaritan at the scene of an accident?
1. Seek consent from the injured party before rendering assistance.
2. Implement every critical-care intervention necessary to sustain life.
3. Stay at the scene until another qualified person takes over responsibility.
4. Insist on helping because a nurse is the best-qualified person to provide care.

13. A faculty member of a nursing program is conducting an informational session for potential nursing students. Which information about licensure to practice nursing upon completion of a nursing program should the faculty member include in the session?
1. "It is a responsibility of the American Nurses Association."
2. "It is granted on graduation from a nursing program."
3. "It is approved by the National League for Nursing."
4. "It is required by law in each individual state."

14. When considering legal issues the word *contract* is to *liable* as *standard* is to which word?
1. Rights
2. Negligence
3. Malpractice
4. Accountability

15. An anxious patient repeatedly uses the call bell to get the nurse to come to the room. Finally the nurse says to the patient, "If you keep ringing, there will come a time I won't answer your bell." Which legal term is related to this statement?
1. Slander
2. Battery
3. Assault
4. Libel

16. A nurse is informed that a credentialing team has arrived and is in the process of assessing the quality of care delivered at the hospital. Employees who are reviewers of which one of the following organizations are associated with the credentialing of hospitals?
    1. The Joint Commission
    2. National League for Nursing
    3. American Nurses Association
    4. National Council Licensure Examination

17. A nurse changes a patient's dry sterile dressing. How is the nurse functioning when performing this task?
    1. Interdependently
    2. Collaboratively
    3. Independently
    4. Dependently

18. A nurse must administer a medication. Which should the nurse do **first**?
    1. Verify the prescription for accuracy.
    2. Check the patient's identification armband.
    3. Ensure the medication is in the medication cart.
    4. Determine the appropriateness of the prescribed medication.

19. When choosing a nursing school in the United States that awards an associate degree, a future student nurse should consider schools that have met the standards of nursing education established by which organization?
    1. National League for Nursing Accrediting Commission
    2. North American Nursing Diagnosis Association
    3. Sigma Theta Tau International
    4. American Nurses Association

20. A patient's diet order is "clear liquids to regular as tolerated." How is the nurse functioning when progressing the patient's diet to full liquid?
    1. Dependently
    2. Independently
    3. Collaboratively
    4. Interdependently

21. Who is primarily protected by the licensure of Registered Professional Nurses?
    1. Nurses
    2. Patients
    3. Common law
    4. Health-care agencies

22. Which factor is unique to malpractice when comparing negligence and malpractice?
    1. The action did not meet standards of care.
    2. The inappropriate care is an act of commission.
    3. There is harm to the patient as a result of the care.
    4. There is a contractual relationship between the nurse and patient.

23. A nurse completes an Incident Report after a patient falls while getting out of bed unassisted. Which is the purpose of this report?
    1. Ensure that all parties have an opportunity to document what happened.
    2. Help establish who is responsible for the incident.
    3. Make data available for quality-control analysis.
    4. Document the incident on the patient's chart.

24. How is the nurse functioning when administering a drug that has prn as part of the prescription?
    1. Collegially
    2. Dependently
    3. Independently
    4. Interdependently

25. Which is the main role of the American Nurses Association?
1. Establish standards of nursing practice.
2. Recognize academic achievement in nursing.
3. Monitor educational institutions granting degrees in nursing.
4. Prepare nurses to become members of the nursing profession.

26. A nurse says, "If you do not let me do this dressing change, I will not let you eat dinner with the other residents in the dining room." Which legal term is related to this statement?
1. Battery
2. Assault
3. Negligence
4. Malpractice

27. For which are state legislatures responsible?
1. Standardized care plans
2. Enactment of Nurse Practice Acts
3. Accreditation of educational nursing programs
4. Certification in specialty areas of nursing practice

28. Nursing practice is influenced by the doctrine of *respondeat superior*. Which is the basic concept related to this theory of liability?
1. Nurses must respond to the Supreme Court when they commit acts of malpractice.
2. Health-care facilities are responsible for the negligent actions of the nurses whom they employ.
3. Nurses are responsible for their actions when they have contractual relationships with patients.
4. The laws absolve nurses from being sued for negligence if they provide inappropriate care at the scene of an accident.

29. When attempting to administer a 10 p.m. sleeping medication, the nurse assesses that the patient appears to be asleep. Which should the nurse do?
1. Withhold the drug
2. Notify the primary health-care provider
3. Awaken the patient to administer the drug
4. Administer it later if the patient awakens during the night

30. Which is the primary purpose of the American Nurses Association (ANA) Standards of Clinical Nursing Practice?
1. Establish criteria for quality practice.
2. Define the philosophy of nursing practice.
3. Identify the legal definition of nursing practice.
4. Determine educational standards for nursing practice.

31. Which of the following patients requires a co-signature for a valid consent for surgery?
1. 15-year-old mother whose infant requires exploratory surgery
2. 40-year-old resident in a home for developmentally disabled adults
3. 90-year-old adult who wants more information about the risks of surgery
4. 50-year-old unconscious trauma victim who needs insertion of a chest tube

32. A patient living in Oregon has been receiving hospice care in the home. One day the patient tells the nurse, "Dying takes forever. I hate it that I am a burden to my family. I can't stand this anymore. Can you help me end my life?" The nurse's personal ethical values do not include complying with this patient's request. Which is the nurse's **best** response?
1. "I will inform your primary health-care provider of your desire to die."
2. "Your family members probably do not consider you a burden."
3. "I can't help you because I do not believe in assisted suicide."
4. "Let's talk a little more about your wanting to die."

33. A nurse working in a hospital administers a medication to the wrong patient and is sued by the patient. Under contract law which liability occurs when the hospital is additionally identified as a defendant in the legal action? **Select all that apply.**
1. _____Vicarious liability
2. _____*Borrowed servant*
3. _____*Captain of the ship*
4. _____*Respondeat superior*
5. _____Quasi-intentional tort

34. A student nurse about to graduate is actively developing a personal ethical foundation for nursing practice. Place the following actions in the order in which they should progress.
1. Clarify personal values and beliefs.
2. Identify ethical issues when working.
3. Identify a personal ethical foundation.
4. Work continuously to improve ethical decision-making abilities.
5. Integrate one's personal ethical foundation within the ethics of the profession.

Answer: _______________

35. A patient sustained a serious injury as a result of malpractice by a nurse. Several legal elements must be met to prove the nurse committed malpractice in a civil suit. Which statements are associated with the element of causation? **Select all that apply.**
1. _____A nurse-patient relationship existed between the nurse and the patient.
2. _____A nurse's omission or commission of an act failed to meet standards of care.
3. _____A nurse's action or inaction was the immediate reason for the plaintiff's injury.
4. _____A nurse should have known that the action or inaction could result in harm or injury to the patient.
5. _____A nurse's action or inaction that did not meet a standard of care resulted in a patient experiencing pain, suffering, and disability.

36. A patient is scheduled to have surgery, and informed consent is to be obtained. Place the following steps in the order in which they should be performed.
1. The patient is willing to sign the consent voluntarily.
2. The patient signs the consent in the presence of the nurse.
3. The nurse determines that the patient is alert and competent to give consent.
4. The primary health-care provider informs the patient of the risks and benefits of the procedure.

Answer: _______________________

37. Identify the actions that are examples of slander. **Select all that apply.**
1. _____Volunteer telling another volunteer a patient's age
2. _____Nurse explaining to a patient that another nurse is incompetent
3. _____Personal care assistant sharing information about a patient with another patient
4. _____Unit manager documenting a nurse's medication error in a performance appraisal
5. _____Housekeeper who is angry at a nurse falsely telling another staff member that the nurse uses cocaine

38. An older adult male is admitted to the hospital after sustaining a brain attack (cerebrovascular accident, stroke). Intravenous fluids, resuscitative medications, and mechanical ventilation are instituted in the emergency department. Eventually, testing indicates absence of brain functions. A nurse interviews the patient's son and daughter and reviews the patient's advanced directives. Legally, which is the **most** likely outcome in this scenario?

1. The son will request that life-sustaining interventions be stopped.
2. The daughter will legally be able prevent the withdrawal of medical interventions.
3. The nurse should refer this situation to the agency's ethics committee for consideration.
4. The primary health-care provider should concur with another health-care provider to arrive at a course of action.

Interview With Patient's Daughter
Patient's daughter stated "I love my dad and I don't want him to die." Daughter indicated that she has been the person caring for her father when he is ill and stated that she will do everything she can to keep her dad alive.

Interview With Patient's Son
Patient's son stated "I love my dad too but if there is no hope for recovery why are we doing all these things? What is the point?" Son indicated that he knows that he and his sister disagree on what should be done.

Patient's Advance Directives
The patient's Health Care Proxy identifies the son as his representative.

39. A student nurse is about to graduate from an accredited nursing program. Which does the student nurse understand are actions **unrelated** to a state Nurse Practice Act? **Select all that apply.**

1. _____Setting guidelines for nurses' salaries in the state
2. _____Establishing reciprocity for licensure between states
3. _____Determining minimum requirements to be licensed as a nurse
4. _____Maintaining a list of nurses who can legally practice in the state
5. _____Providing legal counsel for a nurse who is being sued for malpractice

40. A primary health-care provider asks a nurse to witness informed consents by several patients. Which patients identified by the nurse are **unable** to give an informed consent for surgery? **Select all that apply.**

1. _____16-year-old boy who is married
2. _____50-year-old woman who is confused
3. _____35-year-old woman who is depressed
4. _____50-year-old woman who does not speak English
5. _____65-year-old man who has received a narcotic for pain

LEGAL AND ETHICAL ISSUES: ANSWERS AND RATIONALES

1. 1. This action by itself is unsafe because the patient is confused and the information obtained may be inaccurate.
   2. This intervention ignores the patient's concern. Although this ultimately may be done, it is not the priority action.
   3. **This is the safest intervention because it goes to the original source of the prescription.**
   4. This action ignores the patient's statement and is unsafe without first obtaining additional information.

2. 1. Although documentation of an incident may be used in a court of law, it is not the primary reason for an Incident Report.
   2. Providing a basis for designing new policies is not the primary reason for Incident Reports. New policies may or may not have to be written and implemented.
   3. **Risk-management committees use statistical data about accidents and incidents to identify patterns of risk and prevent future accidents and incidents.**
   4. Although nurses are always accountable for their actions, accountability for the cause of an incidence is the role of the courts.

3. 1. It is unnecessary to call the supervisor in this situation.
   2. Giving the drug as prescribed may be unsafe for the patient and may result in malpractice.
   3. Changing a medication prescription is not within the scope of nursing practice.
   4. **Nurses have a professional responsibility to know or investigate the standard dose for medications being administered. In addition, nurses are responsible for their own actions regardless of whether there is a written prescription. The nurse has a responsibility to question and/or refuse to administer a prescription that appears unreasonable.**

4. 1. **Withholding the medication and documenting the patient's refusal are the appropriate interventions. Patients have a right to refuse care.**
   2. Discussing the situation with a family member without the patient's consent is a violation of confidentiality.
   3. The patient has been taught about the medication and adamantly refuses the medication. Further teaching at this time may be viewed by the patient as badgering.
   4. Notifying the primary health-care provider eventually should be done, but it is not the priority at this time.

5. 1. **Nursing actions must comply with the law, and the law states that euthanasia is legally wrong. Euthanasia can lead to criminal charges of homicide or civil lawsuits for providing an unacceptable standard of care.**
   2. A nurse's beliefs, values, or moral convictions should not be imposed on patients.
   3. Compassion and good intentions are not an acceptable basis for actions beyond the scope of nursing practice.
   4. Nurses as well as other health-care providers cannot legally be involved with euthanasia. In some states in the United States a primary health-care provider can prescribe a medication that can be taken by a patient to cause death. The American Nurses Association, according to its Code for Nurses with Interpretive Statement, indicates that nurses should not participate in active euthanasia or assistive suicide.

6. 1. **The National Council of State Boards of Nursing is responsible for the NCLEX examinations; however, the licensing authority in the jurisdiction in which the graduate takes the examination verifies the acceptable score on the examination.**
   2. The American Nurses Association (ANA) is the national professional organization for nursing in the United States. It fosters high standards of nursing practice; it does not grant licensure.
   3. Sigma Theta Tau International, Honor Society of Nursing, recognizes academic achievement and leadership qualities, encourages high professional standards, fosters creative endeavors, and supports excellence in the profession of nursing. This organization does not grant licensure.

4. The National League for Nursing (NLN) is committed to promoting and improving nursing service and nursing education; it does not grant licensure.

7. 1. A nurse expert can testify for either the defense or the prosecution.
2. A nurse expert can testify for either the prosecution or the defense.
3. The American Nurses Association Standards of Clinical Nursing Practice are authoritative statements by which the national organization for nursing describes the responsibilities for which nurses are accountable. An expert nurse is capable of explaining these standards as they apply to the situation under litigation. These professional standards are criteria that help a judge or jury determine if a nurse committed malpractice or negligence.
4. An expert nurse is not an expert in the law. The expert nurse's role is not to make judgments about the laws as they apply to the practice of nursing.

8. 1. A nurse does not need a primary health-care provider's order to make a referral to a member of the clergy. An interdependent intervention requires a primary health-care provider's order associated with a parameter.
2. When a nurse initiates a referral to a member of the clergy the nurse is working independently. Nurses are legally permitted to diagnose and treat human responses to actual or potential health problems.
3. A nurse can make a referral to a member of the clergy. This action is within the scope of nursing practice.
4. The nurse can make a referral to a member of the clergy without collaborating with another professional health-care team member.

9. 1. A code of ethics is the official statement of a group's ideals and values. It includes broad statements that provide a basis for professional actions.
2. Informed consent is an agreement by a person to accept a course of treatment or a procedure after receiving complete information necessary to make a knowledgeable decision.
3. Nurse Practice Acts define the scope of nursing practice; they are unrelated to participation in research studies.
4. The Constitution of the United States addresses broad individual rights and responsibilities. The rights related to nursing practice and patients include the rights of privacy, freedom of speech, and due process.

10. **1. *Justice* refers to fairness and that all patients should be treated equally, impartially, and without prejudice regardless of individual factors.**
2. The scenario in the stem does not reflect fidelity. *Fidelity* refers to making only promises or commitments that can be kept.
3. The scenario in the stem does not reflect veracity. *Veracity* refers to being truthful, which is essential to a trusting nurse-patient relationship.
4. The scenario in the stem does not reflect nonmaleficence. *Nonmaleficence* refers to preventing harm, avoiding actions that can cause harm, or removing a patient from harm.

11. 1. The nurse is following the primary health-care provider's order to get the patient out of bed. There are no restrictions or parameters in relation to the order. However, the nurse must use judgment before, during, and after a transfer if a patient's condition changes.
2. A nurse does not work collaboratively when moving this patient out of bed.
3. The responsibility to determine a patient's activity level is not within the legal scope of nursing practice.
4. Determining the extent of activity desirable for a patient is within the primary health-care provider's, not a nurse's, scope of practice. Following activity orders is a dependent function of the nurse.

12. 1. Depending on the injured person's physical and emotional status, the person may or may not be able to consent to care.
2. When a nurse helps in an emergency, the nurse is required to render care that is consistent with care that any reasonably prudent nurse would provide under similar circumstances. The nurse should not attempt interventions that are beyond the scope of nursing practice.
3. When a nurse renders emergency care, the nurse has an ethical responsibility not to abandon the injured person. The nurse should not leave the scene until the injured person leaves or

another qualified person assumes responsibility.

4. A nurse should offer assistance, not insist on assisting, at the scene of an emergency.

13. 1. The American Nurses Association (ANA) Standards of Clinical Nursing Practice do not address licensure.
2. When a person graduates from a school of nursing, the individual receives a diploma that indicates completion of a course of study; the diploma is not a license to practice nursing.
3. The National League for Nursing (NLN) promotes nursing service and nursing education; it is not involved with licensure.
4. The Nurse Practice Act in a state stipulates the requirements for licensure within the state.

14. 1. Although patients have a right to receive care that meets appropriate standards, the word *right* does not have the same relationship to the word *standard* as the relationship between the words *contract* and *liable*.
2. The words *standard* and *negligence* do not have the same relationship as the words *contract* and *liable*. Negligence involves an act of commission or omission that a reasonably prudent person would not do.
3. The words *standard* and *malpractice* do not have the same relationship as the words *contract* and *liable*. Malpractice is negligence by a professional person.
4. Liable means a person is accountable for fulfilling a contract that is enforceable by law. Accountable means a person is responsible (liable) for meeting standards, which are expectations established for making judgments or comparisons.

15. 1. This is not an example of slander, which is a false spoken statement resulting in damage to a person's character or reputation.
2. This is not an example of battery, which is the unlawful touching of a person's body without consent.
3. This is an example of assault. Assault is a verbal attack or unlawful threat causing a fear of harm. No actual contact is necessary for a threat to be an assault.
4. This is not an example of libel, which is a false printed statement resulting in damage to a person's character or reputation.

16. 1. The Joint Commission (formerly the Joint Commission on Accreditation of Healthcare Organizations) evaluates health-care organizations' compliance with The Joint Commission standards. Accreditation indicates that the organization has the capabilities to provide quality care. In addition, federal and state regulatory agencies and insurance companies require Joint Commission accreditation.
2. The National League for Nursing (NLN) fosters the development and improvement of nursing education and nursing service.
3. The American Nurses Association (ANA) is the national professional organization for nursing in the United States. Its purposes are to promote high standards of nursing practice and to support the educational and professional advancement of nurses.
4. In the United States, graduates of educational programs that prepare students to become Licensed Practical Nurses or Registered Professional Nurses must successfully complete the National Council Licensure Examination-PN (NCLEX-PN) and the National Council Licensure Examination-RN (NCLEX-RN), respectively, as part of the criteria for licensure.

17. 1. The changing of a dry sterile dressing is an interdependent action by the nurse when the primary health-care provider's order for wound care states: Dry Sterile Dressing prn.
2. In this situation, the nurse is not working with other health-care professionals to implement a primary health-care provider's order.
3. This intervention is not within the scope of nursing practice without a primary health-care provider's order.
4. A nurse is not permitted legally to prescribe wound care. The nurse needs an order from a primary health-care provider to implement wound care.

18. 1. The administration of medications is a dependent function of the nurse. The primary health-care provider's prescription should be verified for accuracy. The prescription must include the name of the patient, the name of the drug, the size of the dose, the route of administration, the number

of times per day to be administered, and any related parameters.

2. Although this action is essential for the safe administration of a medication to a patient, it is not the first step of this procedure.
3. Although this may be done as a time-management practice, it is not the first step when preparing to administer a medication to a patient.
4. A nurse is legally responsible for the safe administration of medications; therefore, the nurse should assess if a medication prescription is reasonable. However, this is not the first step when preparing to administer a medication to a patient.

19. 1. **The National League for Nursing Accrediting Commission (NLNAC) is an organization that appraises and grants accreditation status to nursing programs that meet predetermined structure, process, and outcome criteria.**
2. The North American Nursing Diagnosis Association (NANDA) developed a constantly evolving taxonomy of nursing diagnoses to provide a standardized language that focuses on patients and related nursing care.
3. Sigma Theta Tau International, Honor Society of Nursing, recognizes academic achievement. It does not accredit schools of nursing.
4. The American Nurses Association (ANA) is the national professional organization for nursing in the United States. It does not accredit schools of nursing.

20. 1. This dietary order has parameters that exceed a simple dependent function of the nurse.
2. Prescribing a dietary order for a patient is outside the scope of nursing practice.
3. Collaborative or collegial interventions are actions the nurse carries out in conjunction with other health-care team members.
4. **The primary health-care provider's order implies a progression in the diet as tolerated. The nurse uses judgment to determine the time of this progression, which is an interdependent action.**

21. 1. Licensure does not protect the nurse. Licensure grants an individual the legal right to practice as a Registered Nurse.
2. **Licensure indicates that a person has met minimal standards of competency, thus protecting the public's safety.**
3. Licensure does not protect common law. Common law comprises standards and rules based on the principles established in prior judicial decisions.
4. Licensure does not protect health-care agencies. The Joint Commission determines if agencies meet minimal standards of health-care delivery, thus protecting the public.

22. 1. There is a violation of standards of care with both negligence and malpractice.
2. Negligence and malpractice both involve acts of either commission or omission.
3. The patient must have sustained injury, damage, or harm with both negligence and malpractice.
4. **Only malpractice is misconduct performed in professional practice, where there is a contractual relationship between the patient and nurse that results in harm to the patient.**

23. 1. The nurse who identified or created the potential or actual harm completes the Incident Report. The report identifies the people involved in the incident, describes the incident, and records the date, time, location, actions taken, and other relevant information.
2. Documentation should be as factual as possible and avoid accusations. Questions of liability are the responsibility of the courts.
3. **Incident Reports help to identify patterns of risk so that corrective action plans can take place.**
4. An Incident Report is not part of the patient's medical record, and reference to the report should not be made in the patient's medical record.

24. 1. Collegial or collaborative interventions are actions the nurse performs in conjunction with other health-care team members.
2. Dependent interventions are those activities performed under a primary health-care provider's direction and supervision.
3. Independent interventions are those activities the nurse is licensed to initiate based on knowledge and expertise.
4. **An interdependent intervention requires a primary health-care provider's order associated with a set**

parameter. The parameter, whenever necessary (prn), requires that the nurse use judgment in implementing the order.

25. **1. The American Nurses Association has established Standards of Care and Standards of Professional Performance. These standards reflect the values of the nursing profession, provide expectations for nursing practice, facilitate the evaluation of nursing practice, and define the profession's accountability to the public.**
2. Sigma Theta Tau International, Honor Society of Nursing, recognizes academic achievement.
3. The National League for Nursing Accrediting Commission, the Commission on Collegiate Nursing Education, and state education departments monitor educational institutions granting degrees in nursing.
4. Schools of nursing (e.g., diploma, associate degree, and baccalaureate degree) educate individuals for entry into the practice of nursing.

26. 1. This statement is not an example of battery. Battery is the actual willful touching of another person that may or may not cause harm.
2. This statement is an unjust threat. Assault is the threat to harm another person without cause.
3. This statement is not an example of negligence. Negligence occurs when harm or injury is caused by an act of either commission or omission.
4. This statement is not an example of malpractice. Malpractice is negligence by a professional person as compared with the actions of another professional person in a similar circumstance when a contract exists between the patient and nurse.

27. 1. Nursing team members or an interdisciplinary team of health-care providers write standardized care plans.
2. Every state has its own Nurse Practice Act that describes and defines the legal boundaries of nursing practice within the state.
3. The National League for Nursing Accrediting Commission, the Commission on Collegiate Nursing Education, and state education departments are the major organizations accrediting nursing education programs in the United States.
4. The American Nurses Association and other specialty organizations offer certification in specialty areas in nursing practice.

28. 1. This is unrelated to *respondeat superior*. Negligence and malpractice, which are unintentional torts, are litigated in local courts by civil actions between individuals.
2. The ancient legal doctrine *respondeat superior* means "let the master answer." By virtue of the employer-employee relationship, the employer is responsible for the conduct of its employees.
3. Individual responsibility is unrelated to *respondeat superior*. A nurse can have an independent contractual relationship with a patient. When a nurse works for an agency, the contract between the nurse and patient is implied. In both instances the nurse is responsible for the care provided.
4. This is unrelated to *respondeat superior*. Good Samaritan laws do not provide absolute immunity.

29. 1. This is a violation of the primary health-care provider's order. Drug administration is a dependent nursing function.
2. Notifying the primary health-care provider is unnecessary.
3. Administering a medication is a dependent function of the nurse. The prescription should be followed as written if the prescription is reasonable and prudent. This medication was not a prn medication but rather a standing order.
4. The drug should be administered as prescribed not at a later time.

30. **1. The ANA Standards of Clinical Nursing Practice describe the nature and scope of nursing practice and the responsibilities for which nurses are accountable.**
2. A philosophy incorporates the values and beliefs about the phenomena of concern to a discipline. The ANA Standards of Clinical Nursing Practice reflect, not define, a philosophy of nursing. Each nurse and nursing organization should define its own philosophy of nursing.
3. The laws of each state define the practice of nursing within the state.

4. Educational standards are established by accrediting bodies, such as the National League for Nursing Accrediting Commission, the Commission on Collegiate Nursing Education, and state education departments.

31. 1. A mother may legally make medical decisions for her children even if the mother is younger than 18 years of age.
2. A person living in a protected environment such as a home for developmentally disabled adults may not have the mental capacity to make medical decisions and requires the signature of a court-appointed legal representative. This person could be a parent, sibling, relative, or unrelated individual.
3. Older adults can make decisions for themselves as long as they understand the risks and benefits of the surgery and are not receiving medication that may interfere with cognitive ability.
4. The insertion of a chest tube to inflate a lung is an emergency intervention to facilitate respiration and oxygenation. This emergency procedure is implemented to sustain life and does not require a signed consent if the patient is incapacitated.

32. 1. This statement eventually may be made, but at this time it is not the priority. By this response the nurse is functioning as a patient advocate without violating personal values against assisted suicide. In states such as Oregon, Washington, and Vermont primary health-care providers can order medications that may be used by patients to cause their own deaths; this is called assisted suicide. Certain criteria must be met depending on the state such as 18 years of age or older, a terminal illness with fewer than 6 months to live, capability of self-administering the medication, and specific psychiatric criteria (e.g., counseling, no psychiatric diagnosis, exploration of palliative options). Nurses do not have the legal or ethical right or obligation to help patients die. The American Nurses Association believes that nurses should not participate in assisted suicide or euthanasia.
2. This minimizes the patient's concerns. Also, the nurse may or may not know if this is a true statement; the family members may believe that caring for a dying family member is a burden.
3. Although this may be a true statement, it does not meet the patient's physical or emotional needs. This statement focuses on the nurse rather than the patient.
4. This statement is an open-ended question that encourages the patient to discuss feelings and explore future options including assisted suicide.

33. **1. Vicarious liability applies in this situation. Vicarious liability applies when accountability for a wrong is assigned to a person or entity that did not directly cause an injury, but has a contractual relationship with the person who did cause the wrong. The nurse is still liable for his or her own actions.**
2. A *borrowed servant* does not apply to this situation. A *borrowed servant* applies when an employer directs a nurse to work for a second employer (e.g., agency nurse); the second employer is held accountable for the nurse's actions.
3. The liability of *Captain of the ship* applies in this situation. The liability of *Captain of the ship* occurs when a health-care provider is held liable for a nurse who is working under the direction of the health-care provider. The nurse is still liable for his or her own actions.
4. *Respondeat superior* refers to "Let the master answer" and applies in this situation. When an agency hires a nurse, the nurse functions as a representative of the institution and must perform within its policies and procedures; the hospital is responsible for the actions of the nurse. The nurse is still liable for his or her own actions.
5. A quasi-intentional tort is not related to this situation. A quasi-intentional tort is making false statements, verbally (slander) or in writing (libel), about another person that harm the person's reputation or hold the person up to ridicule or contempt.

34. **1. A nurse must know oneself before helping others. The first step is to identify and explore personal values and beliefs.**
3. Once values and beliefs are explored, then a basis for an ethical foundation of nursing practice can be identified for oneself.

5. After a nurse identifies a personal ethical foundation, it should be compared to the ethics of the nursing profession (American Nurses Association Code of Ethics). This ensures that the nurse works within the standards of the nursing profession.
2. Identifying ethical issues when working in the nursing profession facilitates nursing actions that preserve personal integrity while meeting the needs of patients without imposing personal values or beliefs onto patients or their family members.
4. A nurse's ethical decision-making abilities should never remain static. These abilities grow as one matures within the profession and as a variety of factors (e.g., new technology, evolving social policy) influence one's ethical foundation.

35. 1. This statement reflects the element of *duty*, not *causation*. The element of duty is met when a nurse has a legal obligation to provide nursing care to the patient.
2. This statement reflects the element of *breach of duty*, not *causation*. The element of breach of duty is met when a nurse's action or inaction fails to meet standards of care established by a job description, agency policy or procedures, the state nurse practice act, and standards established by professional organizations.
3. *Causation* relates to malpractice when a patient's injury is directly the result of a nurse's action or inaction (proximate cause).
4. *Causation* relates to malpractice when a nurse should have known that an action or inaction that is a breach of a nursing standard could result in harm or injury to a patient (foreseeability).
5. This statement reflects the element of *damages*, not *causation*. The element of damages is met when the plaintiff proves that physical, emotional, or financial harm or injury was the result of a standard of care not being met.

36. 4. It is the responsibility of the primary health-care provider to include all the information necessary to make a knowledgeable decision. Patients have a legal right to have adequate and accurate information to make informed decisions.
3. Patients must be competent to sign a consent form. The patient must be alert, competent, and in touch with reality. Confused, sedated, unconscious, or minor patients may not give consent. Minor patients who are married, parents, emancipated, or serving in the United States military can provide a legal consent.
1. Patients must give their consent voluntarily and without coercion.
2. The health-care provider witnessing the signing of the consent must ensure that the signature is genuine.

37. 1. This is a violation of the patient's right to confidentiality, not slander.
2. This is an example of slander. Slander is a false spoken statement resulting in damage to a person's character or reputation.
3. This is a violation of the patient's right to confidentiality, not slander.
4. This is not slander because it is a written, not spoken, statement and it documents true, not false, information.
5. This is an example of slander. It is a malicious, false statement that may damage the nurse's reputation.

38. 1. The son by law, as a result of the patient's Health Care Proxy, can make health-care decisions for his father, including withdrawing all life-sustaining interventions.
2. The daughter lacks legal authority to act on behalf of her father.
3. This is unnecessary. Legally, this situation is not an ethical dilemma.
4. This is unnecessary. There are legal documents that will dictate the future course of action.

39. 1. The salary of nurses is determined through negotiations between nurses or their representatives, such as a union or a professional nursing organization, and the representatives of the agency for which they work.
2. A state's Nurse Practice Act determines the criteria for reciprocity for licensure.
3. A state's Nurse Practice Act stipulates minimum requirements required for a person to be licensed as a Registered Professional Nurse or Licensed Practical Nurse within the state.

4. **A state's Nurse Practice Act defines the criteria for licensure within the state. However, actual functions, such as maintaining a list of nurses who can legally practice in the state, usually are delegated to another official body such as a State Board of Nursing or State Education Department.**
5. **State Nurse Practice Acts do not provide legal counsel for a nurse who is sued for malpractice. A nurse should purchase malpractice insurance upon graduation from a nursing program or may be provided legal counsel by an employer.**

40. 1. Legally, individuals younger than 18 years old can provide informed consent if they are married, pregnant, parents, members of the military, or emancipated.

2. **A person who is confused is unable to understand the risks and benefits associated with making an informed decision. In this situation a person designated as a health-care proxy or legal guardian has to make decisions for the confused individual.**
3. A depressed person is capable of making health-care decisions until proven to be mentally incompetent.
4. This person can provide informed consent after interventions ensure that the person understands the facts and risks concerning the treatment.
5. **Narcotics depress the central nervous system, including decision-making abilities. This person is considered functionally incompetent.**

Leadership and Management

KEYWORDS

The following words include nursing/medical terminology, concepts, principles, and information relevant to content specifically addressed in the chapter or associated with topics presented in it. English dictionaries, nursing textbooks, and medical dictionaries, such as *Taber's Cyclopedic Medical Dictionary,* are resources that can be used to expand your knowledge and understanding of these words and related information.

Accountable, accountability
Case management
Change theory
Consensus
Controlling
Cooperation
Creative
Delegate
Directing
Documentation
Efficiency
Empower
Feedback
Five Rights of Delegation:
  Right Task
  Right Person
  Right Communication
  Right Time
  Right Supervision
Flexible
Human resource management
Incentives
Job description
Leadership
Leadership styles—classic:
  Autocratic—directive
  Democratic—participative, consultative
  Laissez-faire—nondirective, permissive
Leadership styles—contemporary:
  Charismatic leadership
  Connective leadership
  Transactional leadership
  Transformational leadership
  Shared leadership
Managers:
  First-line managers
  Unit managers
  Middle managers
  Nurse executives
Motivation
Network
Organization
Performance evaluation
Power types:
  Expert
  Influence
  Legitimate
  Referent
  Reward
Preceptor
Primary nursing
Problem solving
Productivity
Resistance to change
Resource management
Role model
Subordinate
Systems theory
Table of Organization
Time management

LEADERSHIP AND MANAGEMENT: QUESTIONS

1. An accurate assessment drives the rest of the steps of the nursing process. Which management function drives effective management?
   1. Planning
   2. Directing
   3. Organizing
   4. Controlling

2. Which is **most** basic for a nurse to have when working in a management position?
1. Strong interpersonal communication skills
2. Awareness of when to be confrontational
3. Knowledge of the role of a change agent
4. Recognition by peers as a leader

3. A unit manager mentors a new unit manager as part of orientation to the position. Which type of power is being used by the unit manager mentor?
1. Influence
2. Coercive
3. Referent
4. Expert

4. A nurse manager considers that there are "Five Rights of Delegation." Which is a right of delegation in addition to *right task, right person, right communication*, and *right time*?
1. Place
2. Route
3. Feedback
4. Supervision

5. Which should the manager do **first** to overcome resistance to change?
1. Ensure that the planned change is within the current beliefs and values of the group.
2. Provide incentives to encourage commitment of participants to the change.
3. Implement change by employing small steps rather than large steps.
4. Use informational power to ensure that goals of change are met.

6. When considering the autocratic leadership style, an "autocratic" leader is to an "authoritarian" leader as a "democratic" leader is to which type of leader?
1. Directive
2. Permissive
3. Oppressive
4. Consultative

7. Which nursing-care delivery model is based on case management?
1. Patient classification system
2. Diagnosis Related Groups
3. Critical pathways
4. Primary nursing

8. Which statement is **most** significant in relation to the concept of change theory in the health-care environment?
1. Stages of change are predictable.
2. Risks and benefits must be weighed.
3. Change in activity results in positive outcomes.
4. Large change is easier to adapt to than multiple smaller changes.

9. Several nurses complain to the nurse manager that one of the patient care aides constantly takes extensive lunch breaks. Which should the nurse manager do?
1. Convene a group meeting of all the patient care aides to review their responsibilities related to time management.
2. Talk with the patient care aide to explore the reasons for the behavior and review expectations.
3. Arrange a meeting with the nurses so that they can confront the patient care aide as a group.
4. Document the patient care aide's behavior and place it in the aide's personnel file.

10. Which should the nurse do to ensure efficiency when managing a daily assignment?
1. Give care to a patient in isolation first.
2. Plan activities to promote nursing convenience.
3. Organize care around legally required activities.
4. Perform routine bed baths between breakfast and lunch.

11. A supervisor communicates expectations about a task to be completed and then delegates the task. Which management function is being implemented by the supervisor?
1. Planning
2. Directing
3. Organizing
4. Controlling

12. A student nurse in the clinical area is given an appropriate patient assignment by the instructor. Which should the student nurse do?
1. Complete the care indicated on the patient's plan of care.
2. Accept the role of leader of the patient's health-care team.
3. Assume accountability for the tasks that are assigned by the instructor.
4. Help other students to complete their assigned tasks whenever necessary.

13. Which statement is significant in relation to the concept of change theory in the health-care environment?
1. Barriers to change can be overcome by embracing new ideas uncritically.
2. Change generates anxiety by moving away from the comfortable.
3. Behaviors are easy to change when change is supported.
4. Change is effective when spontaneous.

14. Which is the major task of a nurse manager?
1. Accomplishing an objective
2. Empowering others
3. Problem solving
4. Planning

15. A staff nurse must solve a complex problem. Which is the nurse's **most** effective resource?
1. Organizational chart of the institution
2. Nursing procedure manual
3. Unit's nurse manager
4. Nursing supervisor

16. When delegating a specific procedure to a patient care aide, the aide refuses to perform the procedure. Which should the nurse do **first**?
1. Assign the procedure to another patient care aide.
2. Explain that it is part of the patient care aide's job description.
3. Explore why the patient care aide refused to perform the procedure.
4. Send the patient care aide to the procedure manual to review the procedure.

17. Which is the **first** thing the nurse should do when planning to apply for a new position within an agency?
1. Review the job description.
2. Provide at least several positive references.
3. Identify if power is associated with the position.
4. Locate the position on the agency's Table of Organization.

18. Which is the **most** important reason why a nurse aide must fully understand how to implement a delegated procedure?
1. Be capable of completing the procedure safely.
2. Be proficient enough to perform the procedure quickly.
3. Have the knowledge to explain the procedure to a patient.
4. Have the correct information when teaching the procedure to another nurse aide.

19. A nursing team leader delegates a wound irrigation to a Licensed Practical Nurse (LPN). It has been a long time since the LPN performed this procedure. Which should the nursing team leader do to ensure patient safety?
1. Verbally describe how to perform the procedure to the LPN.
2. Have the LPN demonstrate how to perform the procedure.
3. Assign another LPN to assist with the procedure.
4. Delegate the procedure to another LPN.

20. A nurse manager is informed that a large number of patients will be admitted in response to a terrorist attack. Which type of leadership style is appropriate to use in this situation?
1. Collaborative
2. Authoritarian
3. Laissez-faire
4. Democratic

21. A nurse manager is experiencing staff resistance when implementing change. Which is the **most** important action by the nurse manager to overcome resistance to change?
1. Identify the reason for the resistance.
2. Restate the purpose of the change concisely.
3. Modify the objectives to appeal to more key people.
4. Emphasize the positive consequences of the planned change.

22. Which is the major focus of leadership?
1. Inspiring people
2. Initiating change
3. Controlling others
4. Producing a product

23. Which factor associated with a manager differentiates the role of a manager from a leader?
1. Vision
2. Charisma
3. Confidence
4. Responsibility

24. Which situation is reflective of the saying "A stitch in time saves nine"?
1. Obtaining the vital signs of patients on the unit during a specified time frame
2. Collecting equipment for a procedure before entering the room
3. Delegating some interventions to the Licensed Practical Nurse
4. Documenting the nursing care given every few hours

25. A Registered Nurse delegates a procedure to a Licensed Practical Nurse. Which is the purpose for delegating the procedure to the Licensed Practical Nurse?
1. Create change.
2. Establish a network.
3. Improve productivity.
4. Transfer accountability.

26. A nurse manager plans to provide feedback to a subordinate who needs a change in behavior. Which is the **first** intervention by the nurse manager?
1. Be assertive.
2. Explore alternatives.
3. Identify the unacceptable behavior.
4. Document the content of the counselling session.

27. Which is the main reason a nurse manager achieves a consensus when making a decision within a group?
1. Explore possible alternative solutions.
2. Demonstrate that staff members are flexible.
3. Facilitate cooperative effort toward goal achievement.
4. Ensure the use of effective autocratic decision making.

28. A nurse manager evaluates the performance of a subordinate. Which management function is being implemented by the nurse manager?
1. Planning
2. Directing
3. Organizing
4. Controlling

29. Which of the following is related to systems theory?
1. End result
2. Linear format
3. Trial and error
4. Cyclical process

30. Which activities does a nurse manager engage in who values the importance of positive role modeling? **Select all that apply.**
1. _____Counseling subordinates who fail to meet expectations
2. _____Holding team meetings to review rules of the agency
3. _____Engaging in ongoing quality improvement activities
4. _____Reviewing job descriptions with employees
5. _____Following the policies of the agency

31. Which premises are basic to the motivation climate of the Theory Y management style associated with human relations-oriented management? **Select all that apply.**
1. _____Employees will exercise self-direction when committed to organizational goals.
2. _____Employees pursue security above other elements related to work.
3. _____Employees generally will accept and even request responsibility.
4. _____Employees must be pressured with discipline to achieve goals.
5. _____Employees seek direction whenever possible.

32. Lewin's planned change theory progresses through phases. Place these statements by the nurse manager in order as change moves through the process.
1. "Let's implement a pilot project next week."
2. "This is a new venture that should be exciting."
3. "I know it may be difficult but you are doing a great job."

Answer: _______________________

33. Which actions are examples of a nurse working independently? **Select all that apply.**
1. _____Giving a bed bath to a patient who is experiencing profuse diaphoresis
2. _____Limiting fluids when a patient is on a 1,000 mL fluid restriction diet
3. _____Assigning another nurse to administer medications
4. _____Irrigating a patient's wound with normal saline
5. _____Applying a warm soak on an infiltrated IV site
6. _____Obtaining a patient's vital signs

34. A nurse who is a member of a quality improvement committee reviews a chart detailing trends of 4 problem categories identified in Incident Reports over a 3-month period of time. Corrective action plans were implemented to address each problem category. After analyzing the chart documenting tends over the successive months of March, April, and May, which problem category demonstrated the most improvement?
1. Falls
2. Medication errors
3. Violations of confidentiality
4. Violations in standards of practice

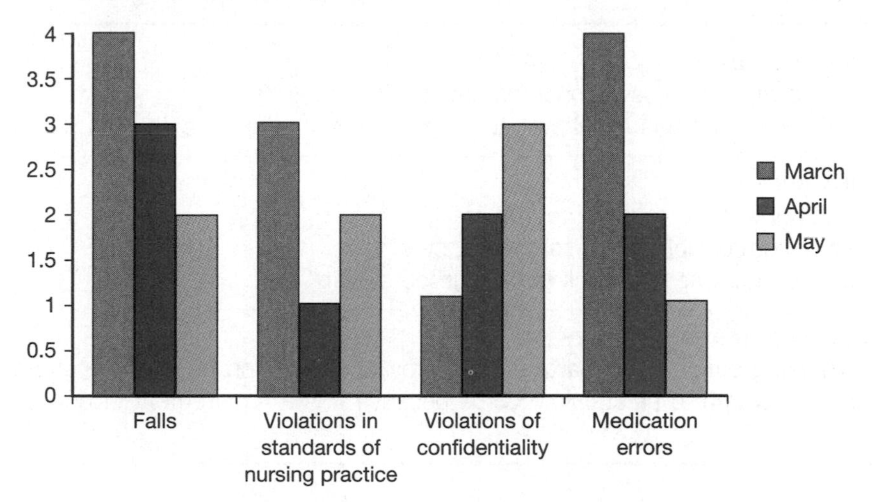

35. A patient is to be discharged from the hospital. Which discharge tasks can be delegated to a nursing assistant? **Select all that apply.**
1. _____Teaching the patient how to measure weight using a standing scale
2. _____Obtaining the patient's temperature, pulse, and respiratory rate
3. _____Determining if the patient knows how to measure fluid intake
4. _____Demonstrating to the patient how to use a walker
5. _____Transporting the patient to an exit of the facility

36. Place the following steps of the decision-making process in the order in which they should be implemented by a nurse.
1. Identify possible solutions to the problem.
2. Gather relevant information.
3. Identify the problem.
4. Evaluate the result.
5. Test a solution.

Answer: _______________

37. A nurse and a nursing assistant (unlicensed assistive personnel) are working together on a surgical unit. Which activities should the nurse assign to the nursing assistant? **Select all that apply.**
1. _____Assessing the results of blood glucose monitoring
2. _____Delivering meal trays to patients who are in isolation
3. _____Explaining to a patient how to use an incentive spirometer
4. _____Changing the linens on beds that are occupied by patients who are on bed rest
5. _____Emptying a urine collection bag that is attached to continuous bladder irrigation
6. _____Assisting the postanesthesia care unit nurse to help transition a patient to a surgical unit

38. The department of outpatient services of an agency is converting from paper charting to electronic charting. The nurse in charge of one of the clinics is responsible for implementing the change on the unit. Identify the **most** significant barrier to change based on the statements by upper-level managers, the nurse in charge, and staff nurses.

1. The upper-level managers have given an ultimatum about the change.
2. The nurse in charge has a negative attitude toward the change.
3. A staff nurse does not know how to use a computer.
4. A staff nurse is anxious about the change.

Nurse in Charge
"Come to me if you have concerns about this change."
"I don't think that this is the way to go but it is something we have to do."

Staff Nurses
"I don't know how to use a computer."
"I feel uncomfortable trying something new."
"Maybe in the long run it will make our job easier."

Upper-level Managers
"The nursing education department will provide classes on how to use a computer."
"We must switch to electronic records because it is a requirement of our regulating agencies."

39. Which tasks should be delegated to a Registered Nurse? **Select all that apply.**

1. _____Obtaining routine vital signs
2. _____Providing discharge teaching
3. _____Evaluating a patient's response to morphine
4. _____Administering a cleansing enema to a patient
5. _____Transporting a patient to the operating room for surgery

40. Based on Kurt Lewin's Change Theory, place an X on the box in which change takes place.

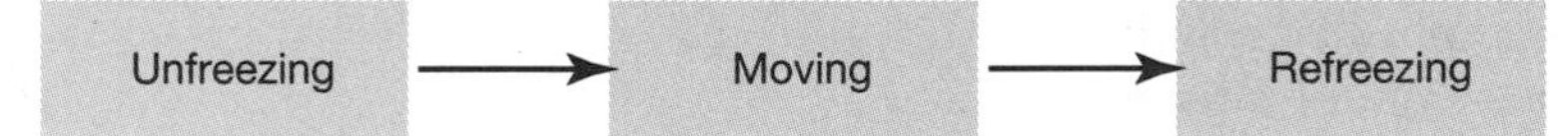

LEADERSHIP AND MANAGEMENT: ANSWERS AND RATIONALES

1. 1. **Effective management depends on careful planning. Planning activities include deciding what is to be done, when to do it, where and how to do it, and who will do it and with what level of assistance. Planning is multifaceted and involves establishing goals, identifying interventions based on priorities, and determining how outcomes will be evaluated. What occurs during planning affects all subsequent steps of management activities.**
   2. Getting the work accomplished (directing) is associated with just one step in the management process and does not drive the process of effective management.
   3. Managing human and economic resources to achieve organizational goals (organizing) is associated with just one step in the management process and does not drive the process of effective management.
   4. Measuring goal achievement, ensuring ongoing evaluation, and implementing corrective action when necessary (controlling) are associated with just one step in the management process and do not drive the process of effective management.

2. 1. **Strong communication skills are an essential competency of a nurse manager. Research demonstrates that 80% to 90% of a manager's day is spent communicating verbally and in writing. Managers must express their thoughts clearly, concisely, and accurately.**
   2. Although confrontation may be used occasionally, it is not as important as a competency identified in another option.
   3. Although knowledge of the role of change agent is important, it is not as important as a competency identified in another option.
   4. Recognition by peers as a leader is not as important as a competency identified in another option. A person generally is promoted to a management position because upper management recognizes leadership qualities. As a nurse manager grows into the role, peers will recognize the leadership ability of the nurse manager.

3. 1. This is not an example of influence power. Influence power is the use of persuasion and communication skills to exercise power informally without using the power associated with formal authority.
   2. This is not an example of coercive power. The leader bases coercive power on the fear of retribution or the punitive withholding of rewards.
   3. This is not an example of referent power. Referent power is associated with respect for the leader because of the leader's charisma and prior successes.
   4. **This is an example of expert power. Expert power is the respect one receives based on one's ability, skills, knowledge, and experience.**

4. 1. The right place is not one of the Five Rights of Delegation.
   2. The right route refers to the Five Rights of Medication Administration, not the Five Rights of Delegation.
   3. Feedback is part of communication, which is one of the Five Rights of Delegation already cited in the stem of the question.
   4. **The one who delegates a task is responsible for ensuring that the task is performed safely and according to standards of practice.**

5. 1. **Change that is consistent with current values and beliefs is easier to implement than change that is inconsistent with current values and beliefs. Values and beliefs are difficult to change.**
   2. This is not the priority intervention. Although incentives might motivate some individuals, they do not motivate all because some people have an internal rather than an external locus of control.
   3. Although small steps are more effective than large steps because they are easier to achieve and once achieved are motivating, this approach is not the first thing the nurse should do to overcome resistance to change.
   4. Although one person sharing explanations with another (informational power) is helpful when trying to change behavior, it is not the most effective type of power to

use when trying to effect change. Another option identifies an action that the nurse should do first.

6. 1. The word *directive* refers to the autocratic, not democratic, leadership style.
   2. The word *permissive* refers to the laissez-faire, not democratic, leadership style.
   3. *Oppressive* is the way some people refer to the autocratic, not democratic, leadership style. There is little freedom and a large degree of control by the autocratic leader, which frustrates motivated, professionally mature staff members.
   4. **The word *consultative* is the word most closely related to the democratic leadership style. Democratic leaders encourage discussion and decision making within the group. The leader facilitates the work of the group by making suggestions, offering constructive criticism, and providing information.**

7. 1. Patient classification systems are not a nursing-care delivery model based on case management. Patient classification systems are designed to assign an acuity level to patients based on their needs for the purpose of determining the number of nursing care hours required to provide care.
   2. Diagnosis Related Groups (DRGs) are not a nursing-care delivery model based on case management. Diagnosis Related Groups are a prospective reimbursement plan in which patients are grouped based on medical diagnoses for the purposes of reimbursing the cost of hospitalization.
   3. Critical pathways are not just a nursing-care delivery model based on case management but are tools used in managed care that are sets of concurrent and sequential actions by nurses as well as other health-care professionals to achieve a specific outcome. They represent specific practice patterns in relation to specific medical/surgical populations.
   4. **Primary nursing is a case management approach in which one nurse is responsible for a number of patients 24 hours a day, 7 days a week. It is a way of providing comprehensive, individualized, and consistent nursing care.**

8. 1. The stages of change are not always predictable. Although effective change moves through three zones according to Lewin's Change Theory (unfreezing [comfort], moving [discomfort], and refreezing [new comfort]), what happens in each zone is not always predictable and change is not always successfully achieved. Change is dynamic and the stages are not rigid.
   2. **Risks and benefits must be carefully analyzed before initiating change. Some change is not worth the risk, because the consequences of failure are greater than the benefits.**
   3. Outcomes of change can be positive or negative. Sometimes well-planned change meets with resistance and the effort to change can result in a loss of credibility, lack of achieving the goal, and confusion.
   4. Small goals are easier to achieve than large goals. Small goals generally are designed to ensure achievement, which is motivating.

9. 1. It is the patient care aide who is late and takes extensive lunch breaks who needs to review the responsibilities related to time, not the patient care aides who follow the rules.
   2. **Recognition of a problem is the first step in the problem-solving process. Once the unacceptable behavior is identified and acknowledged, then the reasons for the problem can be explored, solutions suggested, and expectations reinforced.**
   3. It is not the responsibility of others to confront the employee who is late for work and takes extensive lunch breaks. The employee reports to the nurse manager who is superior in the chain of command of the organization. The nurse manager should meet with the employee. In addition, counseling sessions with employees should be confidential and conducted in private.
   4. This is premature. The nurse manager first should implement an action identified in another option.

10. 1. This may not be possible depending on the needs of patients.
    2. Patient needs are the priority, not the convenience of the nurse.
    3. **Legally required activities must be accomplished because they are dependent functions that support the**

medical regimen of care. Although legally required activities should be accomplished first, many independent actions by the nurse also must be implemented to maintain a basic standard of care and patient safety. Some nursing interventions, which are not essential, can be implemented after the required activities.

4. This may not be possible depending on the needs of patients.

11. 1. This scenario is not an example of the planning function of management. Planning involves establishing goals, designing interventions based on the priority identified, and determining how outcomes will be evaluated.

2. This scenario is an example of the directing function of management. Directing involves getting the work accomplished; it includes activities such as assigning and communicating tasks and expectations and guiding, teaching, and motivating staff members in meeting organizational goals.

3. This scenario is not an example of the organizing function of management. Organizing activities include obtaining and managing human and economic resources and includes identifying the chain of command, determining responsibilities, and ensuring that policies and procedures clearly describe standards of care and expected outcomes.

4. This scenario is not an example of the controlling function of management. Controlling activities use outcome criteria to measure the performance of staff members, identify effectiveness in goal achievement, ensure ongoing evaluation, and implement corrective action when necessary.

12. 1. Although students are expected to complete all planned care, the patient's condition can change or some unforeseen event may interfere with the plan. The student must keep the instructor or preceptor informed about the patient's condition and use the instructor or preceptor as a resource person when the unexpected occurs or guidance is needed.

2. Students are assigned to care for patients for a specific time period and generally are included as members, not leaders, of the nursing team.

3. Students are accountable for the tasks assigned by the instructor or preceptor. As part of accountability, students are obligated to keep the instructor or preceptor informed about the status of the patient, how the assignment is progressing, and whether all interventions are implemented as planned.

4. Students should not help other students unless specifically assigned to do so by the instructor or preceptor. An exception occurs when assistance is needed to ensure patient safety in an emergency.

13. 1. All barriers to change may not be overcome, for example, financial limitations. Before initiating change, barriers should be anticipated and addressed. All aspects of the new idea are best accomplished when critically analyzed.

2. Change causes one to move from the comfortable to the uncomfortable and is known as unfreezing in Lewin's Change Model. It involves moving away from that which is known to the unknown, from the routine to the new, and from the expected to the unexpected. The unknown, new, and unexpected can be threatening, which can increase anxiety.

3. Behaviors are not easy to change even when supported. Most people do not like to function in an unfamiliar environment. In addition, change challenges one's comfort zone in each level of Maslow's Hierarchy of Needs.

4. Planned, not spontaneous, change is most effective because it is organized, systematic, and purposeful.

14. 1. Although planning, problem solving, and empowering others are tasks of a manager, the bottom line is for the manager to accomplish the work of the organization.

2. Although empowering others is one of the tasks of a manager, the major task is identified in another option.

3. Although problem solving is one of the tasks of a manager, the major task is identified in another option.

4. Although planning is one of the tasks of a manager, the major task is identified in another option.

15. 1. The organizational chart schematically plots the reporting relationship of every position within the organization. It does not help a staff nurse identify a solution to a complex problem.
2. The nursing procedure manual is not designed to help a staff nurse identify a solution to a complex problem. The nursing procedure manual contains details of policies relative to nursing practice and nursing procedures along with the purpose and all the steps that one must follow to implement the procedure safely.
3. Generally, in the chain of command of an organization, the staff nurse works under the direction of and reports to the unit's nurse manager. The nurse manager generally is an experienced nurse and is the primary resource person for the staff nurse. The staff nurse should seek guidance from the nurse manager when assistance is needed to solve a complex problem.
4. The nursing supervisor is higher up the chain of command in a Table of Organization than another employee who is the best person for the staff nurse to seek assistance from when needing help to solve a complex problem.

16. 1. Assigning the procedure to another staff member is premature. Another option has priority.
2. The employee may be fully aware of the requirements of the job description and not need to have them described. Even though a task is within one's job description, a person can refuse to perform a procedure because of a reason that is considered acceptable.
3. The nurse must first explore the reason for the nurse aide's refusal to perform the procedure. The employee may have an acceptable reason for refusing to comply. When the reason is identified, then the nurse manager can take an informed action.
4. The reason for refusal may have nothing to do with the lack of understanding of the procedure.

17. **1. This is one of the most important actions by the nurse seeking a new position. The job description provides an overview of the requirements and responsibilities of the role. Job descriptions include factors such as educational and experiential requirements, job responsibilities, subordinates to be supervised, and to whom one reports in the chain of command.**
2. Requesting references protects the hiring agency, not the nurse. This is not the most important thing the nurse should do when applying for a new position within an agency.
3. Although understanding the power of the position may help a person meet the responsibilities associated with the job description, it is not the priority when applying for a new position.
4. Although it is important to recognize where the new position fits into the organization's Table of Organization, it is not the priority when applying for a new position. A Table of Organization schematically plots the reporting relationship of every position within the organization.

18. **1. Safety of the patient is the priority. The nurse aide must perform only the skills that are within the legal role of the nurse aide, understood, and practiced and have been performed correctly on a return demonstration.**
2. Although this may be desirable, it is not the priority.
3. Although this is important, it is not the priority.
4. Nurse aides are trained and supervised by the nurse, not other nurse aides.

19. 1. Providing just a verbal description is unsafe. This does not ensure that cognitive information can be converted to a psychomotor skill.
2. Demonstration is the safest way to assess whether a person has the knowledge and skill to perform a procedure safely. A superior delegating care is responsible for ensuring that the person implementing the care is legally qualified and competent.
3. A peer should not be held responsible for the care assigned to another team member. The Registered Nurse who delegates a procedure to a subordinate is directly responsible for ensuring that the care is safely delivered to patients.
4. This intervention does not address the original Licensed Practical Nurse's need to know how to perform the procedure

safely. This procedure is within the legal scope of practice of a Licensed Practical Nurse.

20. 1. Collaborative is not a classic leadership style. Collaborative refers to the democratic leadership style. Democratic leaders encourage discussion and decision making within the group, which requires collaboration, coordination, and communication among group members.

2. The Authoritarian leadership style is the appropriate style to use in a crisis when urgent decisions are necessary. In a crisis, one person must assume the responsibility for decisions. Autocratic leaders give orders and directions and make decisions for the group.

3. The Laissez-faire leadership style is not the appropriate style to use in a crisis when urgent decisions are necessary. Laissez-faire leaders are nondirective and permissive, which allows for self-regulation, creativity, and autonomy but limits fast-acting efficiency.

4. The Democratic leadership style is not the appropriate style to use in a crisis when urgent decisions are necessary. Democratic leaders encourage discussion and decision making within the group, which takes time.

21. 1. This is essential to overcome resistance to change. There are many different reasons people resist change. Each person will respond to different strategies. There are four different types of interventions to overcome resistance: providing information, disproving currently held beliefs, maintaining psychological safety, and administrating an order or command.

2. Although it is important to state the purpose of the change clearly and concisely, another option is a more important action that can be implemented by the nurse manager to overcome resistance to change.

3. Modifying a goal compromises the integrity of the planned change. All ramifications associated with the change should be explored before beginning and all contingencies planned for so that modifying a goal will be unnecessary.

4. Although emphasizing the positive consequences of the planned change might be done, another option is a more important action that can be implemented by the nurse manager to overcome resistance to change.

22. 1. Leaders can inspire others with their vision and gain cooperation through their persuasion and communication skills (influence power), the respect others have for their knowledge and abilities (expert power), and their charisma and prior success (referent power).

2. Initiating change is the major function of a change agent, not a leader. Change agents are often managers rather than leaders because managers have responsibility for ensuring that the work of the organization is done.

3. Controlling others is a function of a manager, not a leader.

4. Producing a product is a function of a manager, not a leader. A manager is responsible for ensuring that the work of the organization is done, and this often requires the development of such things as a policy or procedure, management reports, and work schedules.

23. 1. Effective leaders and managers both should have vision.

2. Effective leaders and managers both should have charisma.

3. Effective leaders and managers both should have confidence.

4. Managers, not leaders, have organizational responsibility because of their job description. Leaders are not assigned to direct others. They are viewed as leaders by the members of the group because of their experience, vision, charisma, confidence, expertise, or age.

24. 1. Taking the vital signs of all the patients on the unit at the same time is called functional nursing and is unrelated to the adage in the question.

2. This action is an appropriate example of the adage “A stitch in time saves nine.” It means that if you sew a tear when it is small, you need fewer stitches and time to repair it than when it is large. The same adage can be applied to the collection of equipment before a procedure. If the nurse has all the equipment that is needed before

beginning a procedure, less time is used than when forgotten equipment is obtained later. Every time the nurse leaves the room for forgotten equipment, the patient is inconvenienced and time is wasted.
3. Delegation is related to the efficient use of staff and is unrelated to the adage in the question.
4. This example is unrelated to the adage in the question.

25. 1. Delegation is unrelated to creating change. Delegation is the transfer of responsibility for the performance of a task to another while remaining accountable for the actions of the person to whom the task was delegated. Creating change is associated with responding to a stressor that is either planned or unplanned, which results in change that is positive or negative.
2. Delegation is unrelated to networking. Networking occurs when a person makes connections with others for sharing ideas, knowledge, information, and professional support.
3. Delegation allows the Registered Nurse to assign tasks to various individuals on the nursing team who are best qualified to complete them. In today's health-care environment, nursing team members have different levels of educational preparation. The Registered Nurse must take into account the qualifications and scope of practice of each professional and nonprofessional nursing team member and assign tasks accordingly. When this is done, each person's skills and abilities are used most appropriately and productivity increases.
4. The person who is assigned a task is responsible for the outcome of the assigned task. However, the Registered Nurse delegating the task is not relieved of accountability but is responsible for the actions of the person to whom the task was delegated as well as the outcome of the intervention.

26. 1. The nurse manager can provide negative feedback in a manner that is firm without being assertive. Not yielding under pressure (firm) is less confrontational than being confident in a persistent way (assertive).
2. When providing negative feedback, the exploration of alternative solutions is performed later in the counseling session.
3. Problem recognition is the first step in the problem-solving process. Once the unacceptable behavior is identified and acknowledged, then the reasons for the problem can be explored, solutions suggested, and expectations reinforced.
4. Although this should be done, it is not feedback. Feedback is necessary for the nurse to recognize one's offending behavior. In addition, documentation is the last, not the first, step in the counseling process.

27. 1. Exploring possible alternative solutions occurs before achieving a consensus. A consensus is achieved when all, or most, agree or have the same opinion.
2. Consensus, not flexibility, is the goal. However, some members of the group may be flexible and change their opinion to ensure the achievement of a consensus.
3. Cooperation and teamwork are essential for the achievement of any goal. If a consensus is achieved about the value of the expected outcome, people are more likely to work together constructively.
4. Autocratic decision making does not seek a consensus when making a decision within a group. Autocratic leaders give orders and directions and make decisions for the group. There is little freedom within the group.

28. 1. Evaluating the performance of a subordinate does not fall under the planning function of management. Planning involves establishing goals, designing interventions based on the priority identified, and determining how outcomes will be evaluated.
2. Evaluating the performance of a subordinate does not fall under the directing function of management. Directing involves getting the work accomplished; it includes activities such as assigning and communicating tasks and expectations and guiding, teaching, and motivating staff members in meeting organizational goals.
3. Evaluating the performance of a subordinate does not fall under the organizing function of management. Organizing activities include obtaining and

managing human and economic resources and include identifying the chain of command, determining responsibilities, and ensuring that policies and procedures clearly describe standards of care and expected outcomes.

4. **The controlling function of management includes the evaluation of staff members. Controlling activities also include measuring effectiveness of goal achievement, ensuring ongoing evaluation, and implementing corrective action when necessary.**

29. 1. There is no end to a system. Individual parts of a system are interrelated and the whole system responds in an integrated way to changes within a part.

2. Systems do not function in a linear (straight-line) format. Systems are complex.

3. The trial and error method is unrelated to systems theory. It is a problem-solving method in which a number of solutions are tried until one is found that solves the problem.

4. **Systems theory is a cyclical process in which a whole is broken down into parts and the parts are studied individually as well as how they work together within the system. Every system consists of matter, energy, and communication. Because each part of a system is interconnected, the whole system reacts to changes in one of its parts. The concept of treating a patient holistically is based on an understanding of systems theory.**

30. 1. Counseling subordinates who fail to meet expectations is not an example of role modeling from among the options offered.

2. Holding team meetings to review rules of the agency is not an example of role modeling from among the options offered.

3. **When a nurse manager engages in ongoing quality improvement activities, the manager is demonstrating behavior that is expected. The nurse manager also should encourage nursing team members to participate in quality improvement activities.**

4. Reviewing job descriptions with employees is not an example of role modeling from among the options offered.

5. **When a nurse manager follows policies and procedures, the manager is demonstrating behavior that is expected. Role modeling is more effective than telling as a teaching strategy.**

31. **1.** **This statement is associated with the motivational climate of the Theory Y management style. Managers who adopt premises associated with Theory Y believe that workers are responsible and accountable and strive to achieve organizational objectives to which they are committed.**

2. Employees who pursue security above other elements related to work are associated with the climate of the Theory X management style. Managers who adopt premises associated with Theory X believe that workers generally display little ambition and mainly are interested in the security provided with employment.

3. **This statement is associated with the motivational climate of the Theory Y management style. Managers who adopt premises associated with Theory Y believe that workers will be self-directed when a manager assists, supports, and rewards inspired workers.**

4. Employees who require the pressure of discipline to achieve goals are associated with the motivational climate of the Theory X management style. Managers who adopt premises associated with Theory X believe that workers will generally evade work and must be controlled with the threat of punishment to achieve organizational goals.

5. Employees who seek constant direction are associated with the motivational climate of the Theory X management style. Managers who adopt premises associated with Theory X believe that workers will generally evade work and therefore constant supervision is essential for productive workers.

32. **2.** **The first phase is called "unfreezing" and is concerned with identifying the need for change, exploring alternative solutions, and stimulating enthusiasm.**

1. **The second phase is called "moving/changing" and is concerned with creating actual visible change.**

3. **The third phase is called "refreezing" and is concerned with providing feedback, encouragement, and constructive criticism to reinforce new behavior.**

33. **1. Providing hygiene (e.g., bathing, grooming, and oral care) is an independent function of the nurse that does not require an order from a primary health-care provider.**
 2. Providing fluids based on a primary health-care provider's order is a dependent, not independent, function of the nurse.
 3. Delegating tasks within the scope of nursing practice is an independent function of the nurse and does not require a primary health-care provider's order.
 4. Wound care is a dependent function of the nurse and requires a primary health-care provider's order.
 5. Applying heat requires a primary health-care provider's order and is a dependent function of the nurse.
 6. Collecting data about patients is part of the assessment step of the nursing process and is an independent function of the nurse.

34. 1. Although *Falls* demonstrate a downward trend of the number of falls from 4 in March, to 3 in April, and to 2 in May, another category demonstrates a greater degree of improvement.
 2. *Medication errors* demonstrate the most improvement in decreasing errors from 4 in March, to 2 in April, and to 1 in May. This demonstrates the most significant downward trend of the number of events for all 4 categories.
 3. *Violations of confidentiality* demonstrate an increase in the number of events from 1 in March, to 2 in April, and 3 in May. This is a serious concern because the number of events progressively increased in spite of the implementation of a corrective action plan.
 4. *Violations in standards of nursing practice* initially demonstrate an improvement in the number of violations from 3 in March to 1 in April; however, the number increased to 2 in May. This demonstrates a lesser degree of improvement than another category.

35. 1. Teaching a patient how to obtain a body weight requires the knowledge and judgment of a Registered Nurse. Teaching requires a complex level of interaction with the patient, problem solving, and innovation in the form of an individually designed teaching plan of care that addresses the specific learning needs of the patient. In addition, the outcome is unpredictable and it has the potential to cause harm if the skill is taught incorrectly.
 2. Obtaining vital signs can be delegated to a nursing assistant because it is not a complex task. It requires simple problem-solving skills and a simple level of interaction with the patient. Although this task has the potential to cause harm if the critical elements of the skill are not implemented appropriately, it is within the scope of practice of an unlicensed nursing assistant. It does not require the more advanced competencies of a Registered Nurse.
 3. Assessing a patient's level of understanding is a complex task that requires knowledge and judgment and is within the scope of practice of a Registered Nurse. This task requires a complex level of interaction with the patient, problem solving, and innovation in the form of an individually designed teaching plan of care that addresses the specific learning needs of the patient.
 4. Teaching a patient how to use a walker requires the knowledge and judgment of a Registered Nurse. Teaching requires a complex level of interaction with the patient, problem solving, and innovation in the form of an individually designed teaching plan of care that addresses the specific learning needs of the patient. In addition, the outcome is unpredictable and it has the potential to cause harm if the skill is taught incorrectly.
 5. Transporting a patient to the exit of the facility is within the scope of practice of a nursing assistant. Nursing assistants are taught how to transport and ambulate patients safely.

36. **3. The first step in the decision-making process is defining and describing the problem.**
 2. The second step in the decision-making process is gathering significant information associated with the problem.
 1. The third step of the decision-making process is identifying promising strategies to resolve the problem.

5. The fourth step of the decision-making process is implementing an action to address the problem.

4. The fifth step of the decision-making process is evaluating the results by comparing the actual outcomes to the expected outcomes of the employed solution to the problems.

37\. 1. Monitoring a blood glucose level is a procedure that requires the skill of a licensed nurse.

2. Delivering meal trays to patients who are in isolation is within the scope of practice of unlicensed assistive personnel. Unlicensed assistive personnel are taught how to use personal protective equipment.

3\. Patient teaching is within the legal scope of a licensed nurse, not unlicensed assistive personnel.

4. Changing the linens on beds that are occupied by patients who are on bed rest is within the scope of practice of unlicensed assistive personnel. The activity is simple and repetitive.

5. Emptying and recording the volume of output collected from a urine collection bag is within the legal role of unlicensed assistive personnel. The nurse will then calculate the volume of urine by deducting the volume of irrigating solution instilled from the total output. Calculating the actual urine output is an assessment that requires the skill of a licensed nurse.

6\. The postanesthesia care unit (PACU) nurse should be assisted by the primary nurse responsible for the care of the patient. In addition, the PACU nurse must provide a thorough report of the patient's status and important information that the primary nurse should know to care for the patient safely and adequately.

38\. 1. An ultimatum can be viewed as a challenge, requirement, stipulation, or demand. The need to convert from paper charting to electronic charting is a requirement of the facility's regulating agencies. The upper-level managers identified the change that must be made and the purpose for the change, which is reasonable. The upper-level managers will be providing classes to assist the nurses in achieving this change, which demonstrates support for the nurses.

2. Although the nurse in charge appears to be supportive in stating "Come to me if you have concerns about this change," it is better to discuss initial concerns as a group. Specific concerns can be addressed individually later. The statement "I don't think that this is the way to go but it is something we have to do" is a personal attitude that sets a negative tone regarding the change that ultimately may be destructive to achieving the goal of converting from paper charting to electronic charting.

3\. Change may require the learning of new skills. The staff nurse's statement "I don't know how to use a computer" is an issue that must be addressed. The upper-level managers have indicated that the nursing education department will provide classes on how to use a computer.

4\. Change can precipitate anxiety because it involves the process of transforming, modifying, or doing something different. Anxiety is related to that which is unknown. Therefore, goals and objectives must be identified and educational classes provided to help the staff nurses achieve the conversion from paper charting to electronic charting. The upper-level managers will be providing classes to assist the nurses in achieving this change, which demonstrates support for the nurses.

39\. 1. Taking routine vital signs is not complex, has little potential for harm, requires only simple problem-solving skills, involves a simple level of interaction with the patient, and is within the scope of practice of an unlicensed nursing assistant. It requires the more advanced competencies of a Registered Nurse only when previous vital signs have been outside the expected range, the patient is unstable, or the patient is transferred from one service/unit to another.

2. Discharge teaching requires the knowledge and judgment of a Registered Nurse. It requires synthesizing and summarizing information as well as coordinating a variety of community health-care services to meet patient needs.

3. Evaluation requires the knowledge and judgment of a Registered Nurse. The skill of evaluation requires reassessing, synthesizing and analyzing data,

determining significance of data, and diagnosing and responding to the data. In addition, it involves an unpredictable outcome and requires problem solving that may call for innovation in the form of an individually designed plan of care to address the patient's need for pain relief if pain is still being experienced.

4. Administering an enema is not a complex task. It requires simple problem-solving skills, involves a predictable outcome, and employs a simple level of interaction with the patient. Although this task has the potential to cause harm if the critical elements of the skill are not implemented, it is within the scope of practice of an unlicensed nursing assistant. It does not require the more advanced competencies of a Registered Nurse.
5. Transporting a patient is not a complex task. It requires simple problem-solving skills and involves a predictable outcome and a simple level of interaction with the patient. Although this task has the potential to cause harm if the critical elements of the skill are not implemented, it is within the scope of practice of an unlicensed nursing assistant. It does not require the more advanced competencies of a Registered Nurse.

40. **Change takes place when one is moved out of one's comfort zone and into a discomfort zone. The moving stage causes discomfort as goals and objectives are developed and solutions are implemented. Unfreezing occurs before one enters into the moving stage. Unfreezing is the stage where one is aware of a problem and deciding whether or not improvement is possible. During unfreezing one is still within one's comfort zone. Refreezing is the stage where the change becomes a part of the work setting and environment. A new comfort zone is developed as one becomes familiar with the change and incorporates the change into daily practice.**

Health-Care Delivery

KEYWORDS

The following words include nursing/medical terminology, concepts, principles, and information relevant to content specifically addressed in the chapter or associated with topics presented in it. English dictionaries, nursing textbooks, and medical dictionaries, such as *Taber's Cyclopedic Medical Dictionary,* are resources that can be used to expand your knowledge and understanding of these words and related information.

Acuity
Advocate
Baby boomers
Burnout
Career ladder
Case management, case manager
Continuity of care
Cost containment
Counselor
Critical pathways
Demographics
Diagnosis Related Groups (DRGs)
Functional nursing
Health-care team members:
- Activity Therapist
- Certified Social Worker
- Clinical Nurse Specialist
- Licensed Practical Nurse
- Nurse Anesthetist
- Nurse Assistant
- Nurse Midwife
- Nurse Practitioner
- Occupational Therapist
- Pastoral care provider, clergy
- Patient
- Patient's family members
- Physical Therapist
- Physician
- Physician's Assistant
- Registered Dietitian
- Registered Nurse
- Speech Therapist

Health-care settings:
- Acute care hospitals
- Adult day care
- Ambulatory care centers
- Assisted-living residence
- Clinics
- Extended care
- Home health services
- Hospice (inpatient, residential, in the home)
- Industrial or occupation settings
- Life-care community
- Long-term care nursing homes
- Neighborhood community health center
- Physicians' offices
- Psychiatric facilities
- Rehabilitation centers
- School settings
- Urgent visit centers

Health Maintenance Organization
Levels of health care:
- Primary health care
- Secondary health care
- Tertiary health care

Levels of prevention:
- Primary prevention
- Health promotion
- Health protection
- Preventive health services
- Secondary prevention
- Tertiary prevention

Managed care
Medicaid
Medicare
Multidisciplinary
Patient classification system
Preauthorization
Preferred Provider Organization
Primary nursing
Prospective payment system
Reengineering
Reimbursement
Resource Utilization Groups (RUGs)
Sandwich generation
Third-party payers
Types of agencies:
- Official—governmental
- Proprietary—for profit
- Voluntary—not for profit

Undocumented immigrants

HEALTH-CARE DELIVERY: QUESTIONS

1. Which health-care team member can provide independent health care with third-party reimbursement in the emerging health-care delivery system in the United States?
1. Licensed Registered Nurse
2. Clinical Nurse Specialist
3. Physician's Assistant
4. Nurse Practitioner

2. Which does critical pathways in health care refer to?
1. Educational career ladders for health-care professionals
2. Multidisciplinary plans with predetermined patient outcomes
3. Times during life when certain health problems are more likely to occur
4. Organizations that provide services that progress from acute care to long-term care

3. Which setting is the organizational center of the United States health-care system?
1. Clinic setting
2. Acute care setting
3. Community setting
4. Long-term care setting

4. A nurse is explaining mammography screening to a patient. Which level of health-care delivery service does this diagnostic test reflect?
1. Secondary
2. Tertiary
3. Primary
4. Acute

5. When should a nurse begin a patient's rehabilitative care?
1. When the patient is conscious
2. Once the patient begins walking
3. After the medical diagnosis is made
4. Just before discharge from the hospital

6. A nurse case manager is counselling an older adult patient about resources available to assist with the cost of health care. The nurse should inform the patient which organization provides the majority of the health-care costs for people older than 65 years of age?
1. Medicare
2. Medicaid
3. Blue Cross
4. Blue Shield

7. Which result of reengineering in hospital settings has raised the greatest concerns for patient safety?
1. Decreased hospital occupancy rates
2. Increased acuity of hospitalized patients
3. Hospitals merging with larger institutions
4. Substitution of less skilled workers for nurses

8. A patient is discharged from the hospital 3 days after abdominal surgery because of the influence of Diagnosis Related Groups (DRGs). Which should the nurse performing the discharge teaching be **most** concerned about?
1. Providing for continuity of care
2. Ordering equipment to be used in the home
3. Accepting discharge by the patient and family
4. Ensuring hospital reimbursement for services rendered

9. Together the nurse and patient are setting a goal during health-care planning. Which factor generates the **most** anxiety for a patient with this process?
   1. Role
   2. Values
   3. Beliefs
   4. Change
10. Three hospitals agree to work collectively to provide a full range of health-care services in their neighborhoods. Which type of relationship has been entered into by these hospitals?
    1. Integrated health-care service network
    2. Third-party reimbursement system
    3. Health Maintenance Organization
    4. Diagnosis Related Groups
11. A nurse is planning actions that address a patient's health-care needs. Which statement is important for the nurse to consider?
    1. Health and illness clearly are separated at the middle of the health-illness continuum.
    2. Demographics of the population of the United States are changing drastically.
    3. External factors mainly are the cause of most illnesses.
    4. Most people view health as the absence of disease.
12. Which action is common to the majority of Registered Nurse positions in different settings in which nurses work?
    1. Assisting a primary health-care provider
    2. Serving in an administrative capacity
    3. Developing patient plans of care
    4. Providing direct physical care
13. A nurse is planning a community outreach program about the variety of health-care professionals and the services they provide. Which members of the health-care team should the nurse indicate are the largest group of health-care personnel in the United States?
    1. Social workers
    2. Nurse aides
    3. Physicians
    4. Nurses
14. Which is the **major** factor that limits the overhaul of the health-care delivery system of the United States?
    1. Elected officials who do not respond to the pressure of their political constituencies
    2. Explosion of technical advances within the profession of medicine
    3. Complexity of the problems associated with health-care reform
    4. Resistance of physicians to reform
15. Which is emphasized in the traditional health-care delivery system in the United States?
    1. Health promotion
    2. Illness prevention
    3. Diagnosis and treatment
    4. Rehabilitation and long-term care
16. At the end of a shift the nurse in charge must evaluate each patient in relation to the agency's patient classification system. Which is the purpose of this patient classification system?
    1. Document resource needs for the purpose of establishing reimbursement.
    2. Provide data about patient acuity to help assign nursing staff.
    3. Establish that quality standards have been met.
    4. Identify standardized expected outcomes.

17. Which health-care professional is **best** prepared to track a patient's progress through the health-care system?
    1. Case manager
    2. Primary nurse
    3. Nurse manager
    4. Home-care nurse

18. A nurse is reviewing a variety of surveys regarding the delivery of health care within the United States. Which statement reflects a significant change in the thinking of the general public about concepts related to health-care delivery?
    1. "Institutional-based care will have to be increased as baby boomers age."
    2. "More services must address the secondary health-care needs of the community."
    3. "Individuals can influence their own health through behavior and lifestyle changes."
    4. "Health-care providers should be primarily responsible to provide appropriate health-care services."

19. Which group is the greatest challenge to the financing of health care in the United States?
    1. Undocumented immigrants
    2. Medically uninsured
    3. Preterm infants
    4. Older adults

20. A patient asks the nurse, "What is the difference between Medicare and Medicaid?" Which response by the nurse describes the Medicaid program?
    1. "A retrospective health-care reimbursement program that pays for costs incurred by health-care agencies for the care of the indigent"
    2. "A state program requiring primary health-care providers to deliver care to people living below the designated poverty level"
    3. "A federally funded health insurance program for individuals with minimal incomes"
    4. "A federally funded health insurance program for people aged 65 years or older"

21. A patient is told that preauthorization is required before surgery can be performed. The patient asks the nurse, "What does preauthorization mean?" Which is an accurate response to the patient's question?
    1. "Third-party payers have approved the surgery and the facility will be reimbursed for costs."
    2. "The preoperative checklist has been completed and verified by a nurse."
    3. "Required preoperative diagnostic tests have been performed."
    4. "You have signed the legal consent form for the surgery."

22. A patient is to return from the postanesthesia care unit to a semiprivate room. Which is the **most** significant factor concerning the postoperative patient's potential roommate that will influence the nurse's decision to transfer the postoperative patient to this room?
    1. Emotionally fragile
    2. Able to communicate
    3. In the bed by the window
    4. Physiologically compatible

23. A nurse assists a family to explore the options available to help them cope with an older adult family member who cannot live alone because of progressing cognitive difficulties. Which word **best** describes this role of the nurse?
    1. Teacher
    2. Advocate
    3. Surrogate
    4. Counselor

24. A nurse is examining research results regarding receipt of health-care benefits in the United States. Which group of people who were the most underserved before the Affordable Care Act of 2010 now have the opportunity to receive health-care benefits?
1. Children
2. Older adults
3. Pregnant women
4. Middle-aged men

25. A patient with an infection receives medical intervention and nursing care in a hospital setting. Which level health-care service has been provided in this situation?
1. Emergency
2. Secondary
3. Tertiary
4. Primary

26. Which is the cornerstone of *Nursing's Agenda for Health Care Reform?*
1. A standardized package of health-care services must be provided by organizations within the federal government.
2. Health-care services should be provided in environments that are accessible, familiar, and friendly.
3. Advanced practice nurses should play a prominent role in the provision of primary health care.
4. Nursing must provide for the central focus of the health-care delivery system.

27. A home health-care nurse is functioning as a case manager for a patient recently discharged from the hospital. Which is the **primary** role of the nurse when functioning as a case manager?
1. Coordinator
2. Counselor
3. Provider
4. Teacher

28. Which is the **best** example of an inpatient care setting where nursing care is delivered?
1. Ambulatory care center
2. Extended-care facility
3. Day-care center
4. Hospice

29. Which change identified by the nurse will **most** affect health-care delivery in the United States in the future?
1. Less emphasis will be placed on prolonging life.
2. The proportion of older adults in society will increase.
3. More people will seek health care in an acute care setting.
4. Genetic counseling will dramatically decrease the number of ill infants born.

30. Diagnosis Related Groups (DRGs) were instituted by the federal government mainly to reduce which of the following?
1. Number of professionals working in hospitals
2. Focus on illness and place it on prevention
3. Fragmentation of care
4. Cost of health care

31. Which characteristic is unique to the nurse-patient relationship?
1. Patient's needs are satisfied.
2. There is a social component.
3. Both are working toward a common goal.
4. The nurse is the leader of the health team.

32. A recently licensed Registered Nurse is working the night shift on an active medical unit in a hospital. Which is the **best** way that this nurse can prevent professional burnout?
1. Challenge the how and why of one's role.
2. Get adequate sleep and exercise each day.
3. Clarify expectations, strengths, and limitations.
4. Seek a balance among seriousness, humor, and aloofness.

33. Which intervention is **most** likely to have the greatest impact on decreasing the nursing shortage?
1. Providing stress reduction programs to address needs of nurses experiencing burnout
2. Offering bonuses to entice nurses close to retirement to work longer
3. Developing initiatives to fund the education of nursing faculty
4. Increasing the recruitment of foreign registered nurses

34. A patient receiving a special diet is given a meal tray that does not contain a food requested by the patient. Place the following interventions in the order that they should be implemented by the nurse.
1. Check the dietary manual.
2. Schedule a conference with the dietitian.
3. Verify the primary health-care provider's dietary order.
4. Explore with the primary health-care provider the possibility of including this food preference in the diet.

Answer: ____________________

35. Which are examples of an official agency? **Select all that apply.**
1. _____Department of Health
2. _____Veterans Affairs Hospital
3. _____American Heart Association
4. _____National League for Nursing
5. _____Nonprofit community hospital

36. A nurse is functioning as a direct caregiver for a patient with multiple health problems. Which words are **most** associated with the caregiver role of the nurse? **Select all that apply.**
1. _____Implement
2. _____Facilitate
3. _____Evaluate
4. _____Counsel
5. _____Teach

37. An older adult woman, who was incoherent, wandering, and wearing inadequate clothing for the cold weather, was found by a police officer at night. The woman was admitted to the hospital for dehydration and mild hypothermia. The next afternoon a nurse assesses the patient, interviews the patient's daughter, and considers the health-care services within the community. Which health-care service should the nurse explore with the daughter?
1. Respite care center
2. Home health aide several hours a day
3. Full day older adult day-care program
4. Long-term care facility with assistive living services

PATIENT'S CLINICAL RECORD

Patient's Recent History
Patient lives with daughter and attends a half-day older adult day-care program. She experiences episodes of confusion, generally recognizes her family members, but has issues with judgment. She has not attended the day-care program for the past month.

Patient Assessment
Vital signs are all within expected limits including the temperature, which is 97.8°F; knows her name but does not recognize her daughter or grandchildren; moved to room across from the nurses' station for constant observation because patient has attempted to wander off the unit.

Interview With Daughter
Daughter states her mother's abilities have progressively declined the last several months. "My mother doesn't know who we are most of the time. I am a single mom of three kids ages 5, 8, and 10 and I work full time. Lately she has episodes of not knowing who we are. I was shocked when the police called and said they found her last night. I am exhausted. I don't think that I can keep doing this much longer."

38. Which major trends in health care are occurring in the United States? **Select all that apply.**
1. _____Everyone should have access to quality health care.
2. _____Social issues are taking a back seat as a result of the advances in technology.
3. _____Striving for longevity will take on greater concern than quality-of-life issues.
4. _____Health-care providers control the direction and development of health-care services.
5. _____Individuals and families have primary responsibility for making health-care decisions.

39. A home-care nurse is coordinating the delivery of health-care services for adults 65 years of age and older who live in homes within the community. Which factors about older adults have the greatest impact on the delivery of health care to this population within the United States? **Select all that apply.**
1. _____Live below the economic poverty level, necessitating financial assistance
2. _____Number living long enough to become older adults is increasing
3. _____Suffer from significant cognitive deficits as they age
4. _____Tend to fall, requiring expensive hospital services
5. _____Need the services of long-term care institutions

40. A nurse is a member of an agency's Health Care Research and Quality Committee. The nurse reviews the following bar graph regarding patient satisfaction with the hospital experience after implementation of a 3-month initiative to improve patient satisfaction related to four quality indicators. Identify which quality indicator related to patient satisfaction exhibits the **most** significant improvement between January and March.

1. Satisfaction with educational information
2. Satisfaction with pain management
3. Satisfaction with nursing care
4. Satisfaction with overall care

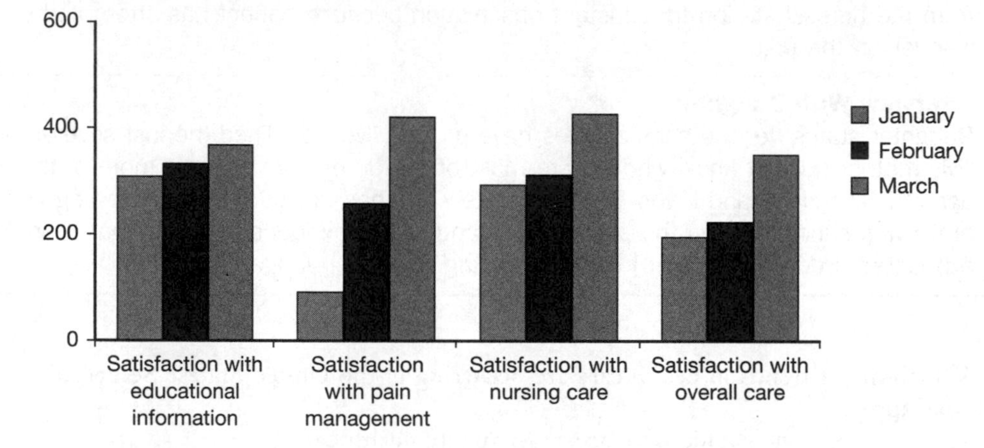

41. Which nursing activities reflect care on the primary level of health-care delivery? **Select all that apply.**

1. _____Arranging for hospice services
2. _____Delivering care in a coronary care unit
3. _____Providing emergency care at a local hospital
4. _____Encouraging attendance at a Smoke Enders' meeting
5. _____Administering immunizations to prevent childhood diseases

42. A nurse is considering the services within the community that can meet patients' activities of daily living and health-care needs. Place these services in order beginning with the one in which the patient requires the **least** amount of assistance to the one in which the patient receives the **most** assistance.

1. An intermediate care setting that provides health-care services to individuals who are not acutely ill
2. An assisted living setting that provides meals and minimal help with activities of daily living
3. An independent care setting that provides meals and housekeeping services
4. A long-term care facility that provides skilled nursing care
5. A subacute unit in a skilled nursing facility

Answer: _____________

43. A nurse is functioning as a patient advocate. Which words **best** describe this nursing role? **Select all that apply.**

1. _____Provider
2. _____Nurturer
3. _____Protector
4. _____Evaluator
5. _____Supporter

44. A nurse reviews the statistics regarding U.S. health-care expenditures published by the Agency for Healthcare Research and Quality, an agency of the U.S. Department of Health and Human Services. Which statistics are accurate and important for the nurse to understand because health-care initiatives must address these concerns? **Select all that apply.**
1. _____Seventy-five percent of the population spends little on health care.
2. _____Five percent of the population incurs approximately 75% of the cost of health care.
3. _____Cancer is the most expensive health condition regarding per-person costs of health care.
4. _____Twenty-five percent of the population has one or more of the five most common chronic illnesses.
5. _____Older adults and disabled individuals who are 25% of the Medicaid population are responsible for 70% of Medicaid spending.

45. Identify which of the following individuals are nursing team members. **Select all that apply.**
1. _____Patient
2. _____Unit secretary
3. _____Registered Nurse
4. _____Licensed Practical Nurse
5. _____Primary health-care provider
6. _____Unlicensed nursing personnel

HEALTH-CARE DELIVERY: ANSWERS AND RATIONALES

1. 1. Licensed Registered Nurses do not receive third-party reimbursement for their services.
   2. Clinical Nurse Specialists are not health-care professionals who receive third-party reimbursement. Clinical Nurse Specialists have been involved in health-care delivery since the 1960s. They are master's-prepared nurses with a specialty in certain areas (e.g., medical-surgical nursing, pediatrics, psychiatry), or they may have advanced education and experience in caring for individuals with special needs (e.g., wound care, enterostomal care, or care of the patient with diabetes).
   3. Physician's Assistants are not health-care professionals who receive third-party reimbursement directly. They work under the supervision of a physician in many different settings and are paid by the physician in private practice or by the organization that hired them. They assist physicians by carrying out common, routine medical treatments, and they have prescriptive authority.
   4. This is a relatively new trend in health-care delivery. Nurse Practitioners generally are master's-prepared individuals who work independently or collaboratively with physicians to provide primary health-care services. Nurse Practitioners work independently under their own license, are accountable for their own practice, have prescriptive authority, and receive third-party reimbursement, depending on the state in which they work. In the states that do not permit this level of health-care delivery, Nurse Practitioners work under the license of a physician who supervises their practice.

2. 1. Critical pathways are not an educational career ladder for health-care professionals. A career ladder is the organization of educational experiences so that professional growth progresses in a planned manner.
   2. Critical pathways are a case management system that identifies specific protocols and timetables for care and treatment by various disciplines designed to achieve expected patient outcomes within a specific time frame.
   3. This statement is a definition of critical time, not critical pathways.
   4. This statement is unrelated to critical pathways.

3. 1. The clinic setting is not the organizational center of the United States health-care system.
   2. The acute care setting is the organizational center of the United States health-care system today. Specialized services (tertiary level of care) and emergency, critical care, and intense diagnosis and treatment (secondary level of care) of illness and disease are provided for in hospitals (acute care setting). In 1991, the American Nurses Association published *Nursing's Agenda for Health Care Reform*, which made recommendations for health-care reform in many areas. The major trend identified as a result of implementation of the recommendations is a shift of the focus of health care from illness and cure to one of wellness and care. If this occurs, the health-care system of the United States will shift from the acute care setting to the home and community.
   3. The community setting is not the organizational center of the United States health-care system at this time.
   4. The long-term care setting is not the organizational center of the United States health-care system.

4. **1. Screening surveys and diagnostic procedures are examples of secondary prevention. Secondary prevention is associated with early detection, early and quick intervention, health maintenance, and prevention of complications. The levels of prevention identify three types of prevention that focus on health-care activities, such as primary prevention (avoiding disease through health promotion and disease prevention), secondary prevention (early detection and treatment), and tertiary prevention (reducing complications, rehabilitation, and restoration and maintenance of optimal function).**

2. This scenario is not an example of tertiary prevention. Tertiary prevention begins after a situation is stabilized and the focus is on rehabilitation and restoration within the limits of the disability.
3. This scenario is not an example of primary prevention. Primary prevention is associated with activities that promote health and protect against disease.
4. Acute is not one of the levels of prevention. The word *acute* refers to the type of care that is provided on the secondary care level of the health-care delivery system.

5. 1. Rehabilitation interventions begin whether the patient is conscious or unconscious.
2. Rehabilitation interventions begin whether the patient is ambulatory or nonambulatory.
3. As soon as a patient is diagnosed with a problem, rehabilitation interventions begin. Care should be present and future oriented.
4. This is too late to begin rehabilitation interventions.

6. 1. Medicare has two parts, Part A and Part B. Most people are enrolled automatically in Part A when they reach 65 years of age. It covers costs if one is admitted to a hospital, hospice, or skilled nursing facility for other than custodial care. Individuals must pay a deductible each year, and those who worked less than 10 years in the United States must pay a monthly fee. Part B covers outpatient care including primary-care provider visits, physical therapy, diagnostic tests, vaccines, and some medical supplies. Individuals pay a monthly fee, a deductible, and 20% of the Medicare-approved amount for some types of care.
2. Medicaid is not a program that pays for the majority of health-care costs of people older than 65 years of age. Medicaid is a United States federal program that is state operated and provides medical assistance for people with low incomes.
3. Blue Cross is a not-for-profit medical insurance plan that pays for hospital services for people of all ages, not just people older than 65 years of age.
4. Blue Shield is a not-for-profit medical insurance plan that pays for care provided by health-care professionals for all age groups, not just for people older than 65 years of age.

7. 1. Reengineering has not reduced hospital occupancy rates. Decreased hospital occupancy rates are related directly to Diagnosis Related Groups and the resultant decrease in lengths of stay. The concerns about a decrease in occupancy rates are not related to patient safety but rather fiscal issues.
2. Reengineering has not increased patient acuity in the hospital setting. Although the increased acuity of hospitalized patients is a real concern when providing for patient safety, safety should not be an issue if a unit is adequately staffed with the appropriate mix of nurses to ancillary staff.
3. Reengineering does not precipitate hospital mergers. Hospital mergers and the resulting reengineering should not impact patient safety if professional practice standards are maintained.
4. Reengineering is concerned with training a less educationally prepared nursing assistant to implement nursing tasks that were formerly associated with the practice of nursing. This trend poses a serious threat to the safety and welfare of patients because tasks requiring the complex skills of a nurse are being delegated to minimally prepared individuals. This is dangerous in the present health-care environment in which hospitalized patients are more acutely ill than ever before.

8. 1. Providing for continuity of care is the major concern with early discharge as a result of DRGs. It requires careful planning to ensure that services, personnel, and equipment are provided in a timely and comprehensive manner and care is not fragmented and disorganized.
2. Although this is a concern for some individuals, if the discharge planner plans early for the patient's discharge, all equipment should be in place before the patient is discharged.
3. Although this is a concern for some individuals, if patients receive supportive emotional intervention and are prepared for discharge from the first day of admission, patients will generally rather be at home than in the hospital.

4. Hospitals are pleased when they are able to discharge a person earlier than the designated length of stay indicated by the DRGs because the hospital keeps the unused portion of the DRG reimbursement.

9. 1. A role is a set of expectations about how one should behave. Although a health-care goal may conflict with a role one sets for oneself, another option has greater ability to contribute to anxiety than one's role.
2. A value is an enduring attitude about something that is cherished and held dear to one's heart and should not generate anxiety. People generally set health-care goals that do not conflict with their values.
3. A belief is an opinion or a conclusion that one accepts as true and may be based on either faith and/or facts and should not generate anxiety. People generally set health-care goals that do not conflict with their beliefs.
4. Change almost always causes anxiety because it requires one to move from that which is comfortable and familiar to that which is uncomfortable, unfamiliar, unpredictable, and threatening.

10. **1. This is an example of an integrated health-care service network. Hospitals are joining networks to decrease costs and increase reimbursement. This is accomplished by expanding the breadth of services while avoiding duplication of services, keeping people within the network, negotiating the price of supplies and equipment, and centralizing departments (e.g., administration, staff education, and human resources), which results in fewer personnel.**
2. This is not an example of a third-party reimbursement system. Third-party reimbursement refers to when someone other than the receiver of health care (generally an insurance company) pays for the services provided.
3. This is not an example of a health maintenance organization (HMO). An HMO is an organization that provides primary health care for a preset fee.
4. Diagnosis Related Groups (DRGs) are pretreatment diagnoses reimbursement categories designed to decrease the average length of a hospital stay, reducing costs.

11. 1. There is no clear separation between health and illness on the health-illness continuum. Each individual's personal perceptions of multiple factors determine where a person places himself or herself on the health-illness continuum.
2. Demographics are changing rapidly in the United States as we become a more heterogeneous, multicultural, multiethnic society. Because of the increasing diversity of the population of the United States, nurses must use transcultural knowledge in a skillful way to provide culturally appropriate, competent care.
3. Internal as well as external factors are the cause of illness.
4. Most people do not view health as the absence of disease. There is no one definition of health because there are so many different factors that impact one's definition of health. Therefore, a definition of health depends on each individual person's own perspective.

12. 1. The majority of nurses' time is concerned with implementing independent and dependent functions within the scope of nursing practice, not spent assisting a primary health-care provider. In most settings, the nurse and primary health-care provider work in a collaborative relationship to help patients cope with human responses to illness and disease.
2. Only nursing management positions contain an administrative component.
3. Nurses work in a variety of settings; however, a component that is common to all settings is the use of critical thinking to develop patient plans of care.
4. Not all Registered Nurse positions include direct physical care of patients. For example, many positions in home care, clinics, industry, and schools focus on case finding, ongoing monitoring of progress, and teaching rather than direct physical care.

13. 1. Social workers are not the largest group of health-care professionals in the United States.
2. Nurse aides are not health-care professionals.
3. Physicians are not the largest group of health-care professionals in the United States.

4. Nurses comprise the largest group of health-care professionals in the United States. There are not enough Registered Nurses to meet the present demand. The Bureau of Labor Statistics Employment Projections 2010 to 2020 released in February 2012 identified the need for 1.2 million more nurses by 2020 to replace retiring nurses and meet the number of new job openings resulting from growth in and aging of the population.

14. 1. Most elected officials recognize the need for health-care reform but generally want to support reform that reflects the desires of their political constituencies. This requires negotiations within the political system that can be prolonged and contentious.

2. This is not the major factor that limits the overhaul of the health-care delivery system of the United States.

3. Health-care delivery in the United States is an extremely complex service industry consisting of public, voluntary, and proprietary businesses with multiple disciplines of health-care workers represented. The system is influenced by federal, state, and local social, economic, ethical, and consumer-driven issues.

4. Physician input is only one factor that may prevent an overhaul of the health-care delivery system of the United States. Although the American Medical Association has a strong political action committee, it was unable to prevent the institution of prospective reimbursement systems that in many ways dramatically changed the work world of the physician as well as placing limits on financial compensation for medical services provided.

15. 1. Health promotion is not emphasized in the traditional health-care delivery system in the United States. However, in 1992, the National League for Nursing predicted that, in the future, health care in the United States will move from the traditional hospital setting to the community with an emphasis on health promotion.

2. Illness prevention is not emphasized in the traditional health-care delivery system in the United States. In 1992, the National League for Nursing predicted that in the future health care in the United States will move from the traditional hospital setting to the community with an emphasis on illness prevention.

3. Traditional health-care delivery has centered on activities associated with diagnosing, treating, and curing illness and disease. In addition, hospitals account for the largest proportion of money spent on health care and employ the largest number of health-care workers.

4. Rehabilitation and long-term care are not emphasized in the traditional health-care delivery system in the United States.

16. 1. This statement does not reflect the purpose of a patient classification system.

2. A patient classification system, or acuity report, is designed to rate patients in terms of high or low acuity; the level of acuity is based on the amount of time and nursing resources that are needed to care for the patient. A patient who is unstable and requires constant monitoring and nursing intervention will be rated a higher acuity score than a patient who is stable and relatively self-sufficient in activities of daily living.

3. Ongoing quality improvement programs are designed to establish whether standards of care have been met and are not a patient classification system.

4. Standardized expected outcomes are established by professional educational and practice organizations, credentialing bodies, and critical pathways, not by a patient classification system.

17. 1. A case manager coordinates and links health-care services to patients and their families at single levels of care (e.g., during hospitalization) and across levels of care (e.g., progression through hospitalization, extended-care facilities, and home care).

2. A primary nurse has total responsibility for the planning and delivery of nursing care to a specific patient for the duration of the patient's hospitalization. Primary nursing is a nursing care delivery system that attempts to prevent fragmentation of care and ensure a comprehensive, consistent approach to meeting a patient's needs while in the hospital.

3. A nurse manager's job is to ensure that the objectives and goals of the organization are met appropriately, efficiently, and in a cost-effective manner.
4. A home-care nurse provides and coordinates health services in the home.

18. 1. Studies and position papers from all segments of the health-care industry indicate the need to provide more health-care services in the community and not the institutional setting. To meet the health-care needs of older adults in the future, efforts have to begin now to provide more community-based support services so that people can remain in their own homes and not have to move to an institutional setting.
2. More services need to address the primary, not secondary, health-care needs of the community. Secondary health-care services include emergency care, acute care, diagnosis, and complex treatment. The present health-care system has an infrastructure that supports the delivery of secondary health-care services. More emphasis must be placed on providing services that meet the primary health-care needs of society, which include health promotion, illness prevention, health education, and environmental protection.
3. Consumers are more aware than ever before that change in their own behavior and lifestyle will have a major influence on their own health status. Public health service announcements, community health education programs, and even television programs and media print materials (e.g., newspapers and magazines) have improved consumer awareness.
4. Consumers, not health-care providers, should be charged with the primary responsibility for providing appropriate health-care services. As individuals or as groups, consumer demands and expectations will have the greatest impact on the delivery of health care.

19. 1. Although undocumented immigrants are increasing in numbers, it is not the group posing the greatest challenge to financing health care in the United States.
2. People who are medically uninsured are not members of the group posing the greatest challenge to financing health care in the United States. There is an increase in the number of individuals who have health insurance as a result of legislation related to the Affordable Care Act of 2010.
3. The March of Dimes identified that 12.8% of live births in the United States in 2005 were premature births. Since then there has been a steady decline to 11.5% as recorded in a preliminary report documenting statistics for 2013. The March of Dimes' goal is to achieve a 9.6% rate in the United States by 2020.
4. The percentage of older adults in the United States is expected to increase to 21% of the population by the year 2040. Because chronic illness is more prevalent among older adults, additional health-care services will be needed in the future. The need for increased services will increase costs.

20. 1. Health-care reimbursement in the hospital setting in the United States is based on a prospective, not retrospective, reimbursement formula. Diagnosis Related Groups is a predetermined hospital reimbursement rate based on a medical problem.
2. Participation in programs providing care to people living below the designated poverty level is voluntary, not mandatory.
3. Medicaid is a federally funded, but state-regulated, health insurance program for individuals with low incomes.
4. This statement describes Medicare, not Medicaid.

21. 1. To maintain quality control and cost containment, third-party payers have preauthorization criteria for surgery that may include requirements, such as second opinions and initial conservative therapies.
2. A preoperative checklist is unrelated to preauthorization. A checklist summarizes the patient's preoperative preparation to ensure that all significant activities and safety precautions have been completed.
3. Diagnostic tests are not related to the concept of preauthorization. Diagnostic tests are performed to identify actual or potential health problems that may influence, or be affected by, the surgery.
4. An Informed Consent is unrelated to preauthorization. Informed Consent is a legal document giving permission for surgery including the procedure, surgical site, and surgeons.

22\. 1. Many hospitalized patients may be emotionally fragile because of the stress of the experience. It is only when patients are a threat to themselves or others that they should not be placed with another patient and should be under constant supervision.
2. The ability to communicate is not a requirement for roommates. A patient does not have to converse with, or be responsible for, another patient.
3. The location of a bed within a room is insignificant. When two beds are available, the choice may be left to patient preference.
4. **One patient's physical condition should not interfere with another patient's physical condition. For example, a patient with a communicable disease should be in a private room, whereas a patient with an incision or an open wound should not be in a room with a patient with an infection.**

23\. 1. The role of teacher is related to helping patients learn about their health and health-care practices.
2. The role of advocate is related to protecting and supporting patient rights.
3. The surrogate role is not a professional role of the nurse. A surrogate role is assigned to a nurse when a patient believes that the nurse reminds the patient of another person and projects that role and the feelings for the other person onto the nurse.
4. **The role of counselor is associated with helping patients and their family members to recognize and cope with physical and emotional stressors and explore options for meeting health-care needs. In this role the nurse must use attentive listening to help patients and family members to make personal decisions.**

24\. 1. **Before the Affordable Care Act of 2010 one in five children lived in poverty and did not have health insurance, and more than 35% of preschool children were not immunized. In 2010 the Affordable Care Act was passed by Congress to address some of these concerns. In 2014 the Affordable Care Act provides for a health insurance marketplace that offers health insurance at a lower cost and with tax credit for families who are economically eligible for assistance. In addition, families can identify if they qualify for Medicaid or the Children's Health Insurance Program (CHIP). CHIP provides comprehensive health coverage based on the state's plan so that parents will not be required to buy a marketplace plan for their children if they earn more than the limit to be eligible for Medicaid benefits.**
2. Although older adults are a vulnerable population, they are not as underserved as a group in another option because of the availability of Medicare.
3. Although pregnant women are a vulnerable population, they are not as underserved as a group in another option.
4. Middle-aged men are the least underserved population of the options offered.

25\. 1. Emergency care is a type of health-care service, not a level of care in the health-care system. Emergency care is a description of one type of service provided on the secondary health-care level in the health-care system.
2. **This scenario is an example of the secondary health-care level of the health-care system. Secondary health care is associated with intense and elaborate diagnosis and treatment of disease or trauma and includes critical care and emergency treatment. The levels of health care should not be confused with levels of prevention. The health-care system has three levels of health care that describe the scope of services and settings where health care is provided: primary, secondary, and tertiary. The levels of prevention identify three levels of prevention that focus on health-care activities, such as primary prevention (avoiding disease through health promotion and disease prevention), secondary prevention (early detection and treatment), and tertiary prevention (reducing complications, rehabilitation, restoration, and maintenance of optimal function).**
3. This scenario is not an example of the tertiary health-care level of the health-care system. Tertiary health care is associated with the provision of specialized services.

4. This scenario is not an example of the primary health-care level of the health-care system. Primary health care is associated with early detection and routine care.

26. 1. Although a standardized package of health-care services is a component of *Nursing's Agenda for Health Care Reform*, it is not the cornerstone of the document.
2. **This statement reflects the cornerstone of *Nursing's Agenda for Health Care Reform*. All people have a right to receive health care, but this right is useless unless the care is easily reached and used.**
3. Although a prominent role for advanced practice nurses is a component of *Nursing's Agenda for Health Care Reform*, it is not the cornerstone of the document.
4. Although this is a component of *Nursing's Agenda for Health Care Reform*, it is not the cornerstone of the document.

27. 1. **The primary role of a case manager is to coordinate the activities of all the other members of the health-care team and ensure that the patient is receiving care in the most appropriate setting.**
2. Counseling is not the primary role of a case manager. When counseling, the nurse helps a patient recognize and cope with emotional stressors, improve relationships, and/or promote personal growth.
3. Providing care is not the primary role of a case manager. When providing care, the nurse is in the direct caregiver role. Caregiving involves identifying and meeting the patient's needs by helping the patient regain health through the caring process.
4. Teaching is not the primary role of a case manager. When teaching, the nurse helps the patient learn about health and health-care practices.

28. 1. Ambulatory care centers are not an inpatient care setting. Although some may be located in a hospital, they are more often in convenient locations, such as a shopping mall or storefront. They provide services such as emergency walk-in care, ambulatory surgery, and health prevention and health promotion interventions.
2. **An extended-care facility is an inpatient setting where a patient/resident lives while receiving subacute medical, nursing, or custodial care. It includes facilities, such as intermediate care and skilled nursing facilities (nursing homes), assisted living centers, rehabilitation centers, and residential facilities for the mentally or developmentally disabled.**
3. Day-care centers are not examples of inpatient care settings. Day-care centers provide care for people who arrive in the morning and go home at the end of the day. They provide care for healthy children or older adults so that significant others can work, or they provide specialized services to specific populations, such as individuals with cerebral palsy or mental health problems.
4. Although hospice services may be provided in a hospital, a nursing home, or a residential hospice setting, the majority of hospice services are provided in the home. Hospice agencies provide multiple specialized services to support the dignity and quality of life of individuals who are dying and their family members.

29. 1. Although this remains to be seen, the explosion in knowledge and technology usually results in treatments that prolong life.
2. **The percentage of older adults in the United States is expected to increase to 20% by the year 2050. Because chronic illness is more prevalent among older adults, additional health-care services will be needed in the future, raising costs.**
3. More people will seek health care in the home and community, not the acute care setting. In 1992 the National League for Nursing predicted that home care will become the center of health care and that community nursing centers and community health programs will focus on illness prevention and health promotion.
4. This may or may not occur because of a multiplicity of factors, such as religious beliefs, unplanned pregnancies, and a lack of seeking genetic counseling.

30. 1. This is not the reason why DRGs were instituted. In addition, the DRGs have increased the acuity of hospitalized patients requiring a lower ratio of nurses to patients, which necessitates the need to hire more nurses. However, many hospitals have not increased the number of nurses because of reengineering and the lack of available qualified nurses.

2. This is not the reason why DRGs were instituted. Although there is a current trend in the United States with more people focusing on health promotion and illness prevention, it is unrelated to DRGs.
3. DRGs were not instituted to solve fragmentation of care. Fragmentation of care generally is caused by overspecialization and caregivers failing to address patients' needs holistically and comprehensively.
4. **The DRGs, pretreatment diagnoses reimbursement categories, were designed to decrease the average length of a hospital stay, reducing costs.**

31. 1. Because of circumstances, a nurse's intervention may not always be able to meet a patient's perceived needs.
2. The nurse-patient relationship is a therapeutic, not social, relationship.
3. **When planning patient care, the nurse and patient work together to identify appropriate goals and interventions to facilitate goal achievement.**
4. The patient, not the nurse, is the leader of the health-care team.

32. 1. How one practices nursing and why one is a nurse are based on enduring values and beliefs. Although it is important to be aware of how one practices nursing and why one is a nurse, confronting, taking exception to, and calling into question one's enduring values are not where the problem of burnout lies.
2. Although it is important to reduce the effects of stress, these approaches do not reduce the contributing factors that cause stress.
3. **When faced with any stressful situation that can lead to feelings of burnout, the nurse must begin with self-awareness and identify personal expectations, strengths, and limitations associated with the job. After the assessment is complete and problems are identified, the nurse can explore options to reduce factors contributing to job-related stress. Burnout generally occurs because nurses are unable to practice nursing as they were taught based on principles and standards of practice. Nurses experience stress because of such factors as understaffing, increased patient care assignments, shift work, excessive mandatory overtime, inadequate support, and caring for more patients who are critically ill and dying. The nurse must employ strategies to manage stress to prevent the physical and emotional exhaustion associated with burnout and not wait until these responses occur.**
4. Although humor may temporarily defuse a stressful situation, it is not an effective strategy to cope with the major issues that contribute to burnout. The nurse should not be distant from the patient.

33. 1. Although nurses are leaving the profession because it is stressful, physically strenuous, and demanding work, it is not the major reason for the nurse shortage.
2. A bonus to entice nurses close to retirement age to work longer is a short-term and limited response to the need for more nurses. Retirement of nurses is not the major cause of the nursing shortage.
3. **Programs to fund the education of nursing educators will most likely have the greatest impact on reducing the nursing shortage. Many nursing schools are unable to accept eligible applicants to nursing programs each year because of the shortage of faculty. The American Association of Colleges of Nursing report on 2012–2013 *Enrollment and Graduation in Baccalaureate and Graduate Programs of Nursing* indicated that nursing schools turned away over 78,089 eligible candidates to baccalaureate and graduate nursing programs mainly as a result of insufficient faculty in addition to other constraints such as insufficient clinical sites, classrooms, and preceptors as well as budget constraints.**
4. Hiring foreign nurses is not a long-term strategy to increase the number of nurses. It will worsen the shortage in their own countries, because the nursing shortage is a global problem, and it will raise concerns regarding effects on salaries, adequacy of education, and quality care here in the United States.

34. 3. **Providing a special diet is a dependent function of the nurse. The primary health-care provider's order should be verified first.**

1. **The dietary manual should be reviewed to determine if the requested food is permitted on the ordered diet.**
2. **If the requested food is not indicated on the diet in the dietary manual, the nurse should collaborate with appropriate dietary resources (e.g., nutritionist, dietitian).**
4. **If the food is not permitted on the diet, the nurse can function as a patient advocate by collaborating with the primary health-care provider to determine if an occasional concession can be made regarding a patient's food preference.**

35. 1. **Departments of health (state, county, city, or other local government units) are considered official agencies because primarily they are funded by tax money. They are concerned with health promotion and disease prevention.**
2. **A Veterans Affairs Hospital is an official organization because it is a part of the Department of Veterans Affairs, which is under the umbrella of federally supported/operated facilities and is financed by taxation.**
3. The American Heart Association is a voluntary not-for-profit organization, not an official organization.
4. The National League for Nursing (NLN) is a not-for-profit organization founded in 1952 to foster the development and improvement of nursing education and services. It is not an official organization.
5. Nonprofit community hospitals are voluntary, not official, organizations.

36. 1. **The caregiver role is associated with the performance of interventions that will help a patient achieve identified goals.**
2. **The caregiver role is associated with facilitating the achievement of goals identified in the patient's plan of care.**
3. Of the options offered, the word *evaluate* is not the word most associated with the nurse functioning as a caregiver. Although evaluation is important in relation to the nursing process and caregiving, it is only one aspect of caregiving.
4. Of the options offered, the word *counsel* is not the word most associated with the nurse functioning as a caregiver. When counseling, the nurse helps a patient recognize and cope with emotional stressors, improve relationships, and/or promote personal growth; it is only one aspect of caregiving.
5. Of the options offered, the word *teach* is not the word most associated with the nurse functioning as a caregiver. When teaching, the nurse helps the patient learn about health and health-care practices, and it is only one aspect of caregiving.

37. 1. The daughter needs more than a brief period of relief from caring for her mother. She is a single mother working full time and caring for three small children.
2. A home health aide several hours a day is an inadequate level of care to keep the patient safe.
3. A full-day older adult day-care program may be capable of meeting the patient's needs during the day. However, the patient also needs supervision during the night, which may be beyond what the daughter can provide.
4. **The patient requires assistance with the activities of daily living and supervision 24 hours a day to prevent wandering and promote safety.**

38. 1. **The Affordable Care Act is a movement in the United States to ensure access to quality health care for all.**
2. Social issues are taking a front, not back, seat as a result of advances in technology. Technological advances and specialized treatments are extremely expensive. Social issues include who will pay for health-care costs, who has access to health care, and who will care for older adults and the uninsured (both of whom are increasing in numbers). In addition, ethical issues are becoming prominent in response to advances in areas such as organ transplantation and beginning of life technology.
3. Although some people strive to sustain life at any cost, most people prefer to seek ways to support and maintain quality, over longevity, of life. The hospice movement, which is increasing, is based on the concept of maintaining quality of life by caring for dying people in their homes surrounded by family and friends and making remaining days as comfortable and meaningful as possible.
4. Educated consumers, not health-care providers, control the direction and development of health-care services.

Citizens are active members of the boards of trustees of health-care agencies in all settings, community organizations have political action committees that lobby government representatives to shape the political agenda, and the consumer movement has demands and expectations; all of these impact the direction of health-care reform.

5. **The patient is the center of the health-care team and has primary responsibility for making health-care decisions. Consumers are more knowledgeable than ever before, have a greater awareness of health issues, and have a desire to be responsible for health-care decisions. In addition, more knowledgeable consumers (patients and families) have made a major impact on the delivery of health-care services in the United States because they have made their opinions and preferences known.**

39. 1. The percentage of older adults below the designated poverty level has continued to decline as reported by the United States Census Bureau. The poverty rate for older adults dropped significantly in the 1970s and has continued to decline to 9.7% in 2012 and to 9.5% in 2013 in spite of the recent recession. Poverty does not have a significant impact on the delivery of health care to people 65 years of age and older living in the community. In 2013, the poverty rate for adults 18 to 64 years of age was 13.6%.

2. **Thirteen percent of the population was 65 years of age and older in 2010 (40.3 million people). The United States Census Bureau predicts that in 2050 there will be an increase to 80 million older adults, accounting for 20% of the population. This is a major factor that has significant impact on the delivery of health care within the United States as the number of individuals 65 years of age and older increases as baby boomers age.**

3. **The percentage of older adults experiencing cognitive deficits varies depending on the agency compiling the research. The Centers for Disease Control and Prevention identified that in 2013, 5 million Americans aged 65 years or older have Alzheimer's disease. It is predicted that this number may increase to 13.8 million individuals by 2050. This is a major factor that has significant impact on the delivery of health care within the United States as the number of individuals 65 years of age and older increases as baby boomers age.**

4. **The Centers for Disease Control and Prevention reported in 2012 that one-third of older adults 65 years of age and older experience at least one fall each year. Falls have become the leading cause of fatal and nonfatal injuries for older adults. In 2012 the cost of medical care for individuals experiencing falls was 30 billion dollars. This is a major factor that has significant impact on the delivery of health care within the United States as the number of individuals 65 years of age and older increases as baby boomers age.**

5. **The United States Census Bureau reported that the percentage of individuals 65 years of age and older residing in a nursing home declined from 5.1% in 1990 to 4.5% in 2000 and to 3.1% in 2010. Although this number declined between 1990 and 2010, the overall number of persons 65 years of age and older living in a nursing home will increase in the future because the population in this age group will increase as baby boomers age. The Census Bureau predicts that by 2050, people 65 years of age and older will double to 80 million and be 20% of the population.**

40. 1. Although satisfaction with educational information improved between January and March, the improvement was not as significant as improvement in another option.

2. **Although all four quality indicators related to patient satisfaction demonstrated a positive trend toward greater satisfaction, satisfaction with pain management increased most dramatically from January to March.**

3. Although satisfaction with nursing care improved between January and March, the improvement was not as significant as improvement in another option.

4. Although satisfaction with overall care improved between January and March, the improvement was not as significant as improvement in another option.

41. 1. This action is an example of care associated with the tertiary level of health-care delivery. Tertiary care is associated with long-term, chronic, and hospice care and specialized services.
 2. This action is an example of care on the secondary level of health-care delivery. Secondary care (acute care) includes emergency treatment, critical care, and care associated with intensive and elaborate diagnosis and treatment.
 3. This action is an example of care on the secondary level of health-care delivery. Secondary care (acute care) includes emergency treatment, critical care, and care associated with intensive and elaborate diagnosis and treatment.
 4. This action is an example of the primary level of health-care delivery. Primary care is associated with activities that promote health and protect against disease. The health-care system has three levels of health-care delivery that describe the scope of services and settings: primary, secondary, and tertiary.
 5. This action is an example of the primary level of health-care delivery. Primary care includes activities that protect a person from contracting a disease.

42. **3. An independent care setting provides personal space (e.g., one-bedroom apartment, studio apartment) as well as services such meals, housekeeping, and van rides to stores or appointments. Individuals living in this type of setting must be self-sufficient, cognitively competent, and capable of meeting their own physical needs.**
 2. In addition to the services provided in an independent care setting, an assisted living setting provides help with some of the activities of daily living such as dressing, bathing, and ambulating.
 1. An intermediate care setting provides health-care services to individuals who require lifelong assistance with the activities of daily living such as individuals who are cognitively impaired or disabled. These settings provide custodial care and function as the individual's home.
 5. A subacute unit in a skilled nursing facility provides care to individuals with an acute illness, injury, or exacerbation of a disease process that requires skilled health-care services but does not require hospitalization to an acute care facility. The services include activities such as occupational therapy, physical therapy, and learning self-care of a newly created colostomy.
 4. Skilled nursing care that must be provided for an extended period of time, frequently for the rest of the person's life, is often provided in a long-term care facility. Examples of patients residing in this type of long-term care setting include people with spinal cord injuries, patients in a coma, patients on mechanical ventilation, and people receiving enteral nutrition via a surgically implanted GI tube.

43. 1. When functioning as a *provider*, the nurse is in the caregiver, not advocate, role. Caregiving involves identifying and meeting the patient's needs by helping the patient regain health through the caring process.
 2. When functioning as a *nurture*r, the nurse is in the caregiver, not advocate, role. Nurture means to encourage, foster, and promote, all of which are components of caregiving.
 3. The word *protector* describes the role of the nurse when functioning as the patient's advocate. In the role of advocate, the nurse supports patients' rights and assists in asserting those rights when patients are unable to defend themselves.
 4. Evaluation is the last step in the nursing process; it involves a determination of whether the patient's goals are achieved. The word *evaluator* is not synonymous with the word *advocate*.
 5. The word *supporter* describes the role of the nurse when functioning as the patient's advocate. In the role of advocate, the nurse protects patients' rights and assists in asserting those rights when patients are unable to defend themselves.

44. 1. Fifty percent of the population spends little on health care.
 2. Five percent of the population incurs approximately 50% of the cost of health care.
 3. This is a true statement about the cost of cancer care per person.

4. **This is a true statement about the percentage of people in the population with one or more chronic illnesses.**
5. **This is a true statement regarding the population responsible for 70% of Medicaid spending.**

45. 1. **The patient is the center of the health team as well as the nursing team. The patient is the most important member of these teams.**
2. The unit secretary is not a member of the nursing team but is a supportive health-team member.
3. **A Registered Nurse is a member of the nursing team. A Registered Nurse provides direct nursing care and supervises other members of the nursing team such as Licensed Practical Nurses and unlicensed assistive nursing personnel.**
4. **A Licensed Practical Nurse provides uncomplicated direct patient care and works in a structured environment under the direction of a Registered Nurse.**
5. Primary health-care providers are not members of the nursing team. They are professional health-team members who have a prescriptive license such as a medical doctor (MD), nurse practitioner (NP), and physician's assistant (PA).
6. **Unlicensed assistive nursing personnel (e.g., nursing associate, nursing assistant, nurse's aide) are members of the nursing team who provide uncomplicated direct care to patients such as bathing, feeding, dressing, and ambulating.**

Community-Based Nursing

KEYWORDS

The following words include nursing/medical terminology, concepts, principles, and information relevant to content specifically addressed in the chapter or associated with topics presented in it. English dictionaries, nursing textbooks, and medical dictionaries, such as *Taber's Cyclopedic Medical Dictionary,* are resources that can be used to expand your knowledge and understanding of these words and related information.

Case management
Community
Demographics
Epidemiology
Health-care reform
Health-care settings:
- Acute care hospitals
- Adult day-care centers
- Ambulatory care centers
- Assisted-living residences
- Clinics
- Extended care facilities
- Home health services
- Hospice (inpatient, residential, in the home)
- Industrial or occupation settings
- Life-care communities
- Long-term care nursing homes
- Neighborhood community health centers
- Physicians' offices
- Psychiatric facilities
- Rehabilitation centers
- School settings
- Urgent visit centers

Healthy People 2020
Holistic
Levels of health-care delivery:
- Primary
- Secondary
- Tertiary

Levels of prevention:
- Primary prevention
- Health promotion
- Health protection
- Preventive health services
- Secondary prevention
- Tertiary prevention

Managed care
Metropolitan
Nursing's Agenda for Health Care Reform
Occupational nurse
Outreach
Population
Primary care
Public health nurse
Quality improvement, quality management
Respite care
Rural
Self-help group
Suburban
Urban
Vulnerable populations
Wellness

COMMUNITY-BASED NURSING: QUESTIONS

1. A family member requests relief from caring for a relative who has a rapidly debilitating malignancy. To which resource should the nurse refer the family member for respite care?
1. Hospice
2. Meals on Wheels
3. Ambulatory care center
4. Alcohol treatment center

2. Which role of the nurse takes on more emphasis in the delivery of health care in the home than in acute care?
1. Coordinating the efforts of the health-care team
2. Delivering skilled nursing care
3. Providing for healthy meals
4. Modifying the environment

3. Which is unique to the home-care setting that is different in the acute care setting?
   1. Patient is the center of the health-care team.
   2. Nurse functions as an advocate for the patient.
   3. Nurse is responsible for coordinating the efforts of the patient's health-care team.
   4. Patient is not discharged until teaching regarding self-care activities is completed.

4. Which action reflects the nurse's attempt to work with family members to explore the nature and consequences of their choices?
   1. Affirming
   2. Mediating
   3. Informing
   4. Interviewing

5. When do nursing activities related to community nursing begin?
   1. On the first contact with the patient
   2. After the patient is admitted to the hospital
   3. At the time referrals are made to community resources
   4. When the primary health-care provider writes discharge orders

6. A nurse must collect information about a community to identify its needs. Which is the **most** significant assessment by the nurse?
   1. The demographics of the community
   2. What the community thinks is important
   3. How many support services are available
   4. Environmental data as they relate to public safety

7. A home-care nurse is caring for a variety of patients in their homes. Which individual identified by the nurse will have the **most** difficult time adjusting to a prescribed regimen of long-term home health care?
   1. Middle school–aged child
   2. Preschool-aged child
   3. Adolescent
   4. Older adult

8. Which is unique to the home-care setting that is different in the acute care setting?
   1. Nurses work more independently.
   2. Nurses require excellent communication skills.
   3. Patients must be taught how to care for themselves.
   4. Patients have needs that require less technical nursing skills.

9. A woman is concerned about her children accidentally ingesting her husband's prescription medications. Where should the home-care nurse teach the mother to keep medications?
   1. On a high shelf
   2. In a locked cabinet
   3. In a medicine cabinet in the bathroom
   4. On a shelf in the back of the refrigerator

10. Who is the **most** important health-care team member in an assisted-living facility?
    1. Occupational Therapist
    2. Nurse Aide
    3. Patient
    4. Nurse

11. A patient's contract for home-care services is about to end but the patient still requires care. On which factor will the continuation of services **initially** depend?
    1. Nursing documentation of the need for care
    2. Retrospective audits of quality management
    3. Patient satisfaction with the care being provided
    4. Presence of a primary health-care provider's order

12. Which factor is essential to the health of a community?
    1. Availability of medical specialists
    2. Individuals having health insurance
    3. Everyone having access to health care
    4. Public Health Nurses working in the community

13. A nurse identifies the health-care needs of the members of a community. Which is the nurse's **most** efficient initial approach to meet these needs?
    1. Involve community leaders to work within the political arena to obtain funding for programs.
    2. Write research grants to explore the community's health needs in more detail.
    3. Design educational programs that address the identified community needs.
    4. Make residents aware of the resources in the community.

14. A home-care nurse is performing an initial patient and home assessment. Which is the **most** essential assessment that must be made by the nurse?
    1. Can the home environment support the safety of the patient?
    2. Is the family willing to participate in the patient's recovery?
    3. Does the patient have the potential for self-care?
    4. Can the patient participate in the plan of care?

15. During the process of performing a community assessment, the nurse invites members of the community to come to a meeting and share opinions and concerns about a particular issue. Which is this method of data collection?
    1. An opinion survey
    2. A community forum
    3. A demographic assessment
    4. An observation of participants

16. Which is **most** important when a nurse works in the home-care setting?
    1. Case management
    2. Discharge planning
    3. Enlisting family support
    4. Modifying patient values

17. A nurse is preparing a patient for discharge from the hospital. Which is designed primarily to provide for a continuum of comprehensive health care after discharge?
    1. Primary health-care providers' offices
    2. Home-care agencies
    3. Urgent visit centers
    4. Respite programs

18. A nurse must conduct a community assessment. Which information should the nurse collect **first**?
    1. General health of community members
    2. Characteristics of community members
    3. Physical environment of the community
    4. Social services available in the community

19. A nurse in a home-care agency is providing an orientation program to a group of newly hired patient companions. Which should the nurse teach them about families in the United States?
    1. Families are groups of people related by blood, marriage, adoption, or birth.
    2. Families are made up of fathers, mothers, and their children.
    3. Families vary based on their structural composition.
    4. Families live in the same household.

20. A home-care nurse is providing care for a family supporting a patient with a chronic illness. Which is the **most** important factor the nurse should teach caregivers who care for a family member who has a stable but chronic illness and is living in the home?
1. Have extra equipment and supplies for emergencies.
2. Plan a daily and monthly schedule of activities.
3. Keep a daily journal of the patient's status.
4. Tend to themselves as well as the patient.

21. Which is a need that falls within the category of tertiary health-care services?
1. Critical care
2. Long-term care
3. Diagnostic care
4. Preventive care

22. A person at home is recovering from an illness that has caused functional deficits. Which support service identified by the nurse will provide the **most** benefit for this person?
1. Hospice services
2. Church outreach program
3. Home health-care agency
4. Meals on Wheels program

23. A nurse is providing information about taking medication in the home. Which is a feature common to **most** containers for prescription medications that should be discussed?
1. Drip-proof tops
2. Unit dose packages
3. Sun-repellent plastic
4. Child-resistant covers

24. A nurse must initiate nursing services in the home setting. Which is an important factor that the nurse must consider to ensure third-party reimbursement?
1. The patient must be able to perform some self-care.
2. The family has the financial resources to pay for the care.
3. Additional family members need to be available for support.
4. Intervention must be ordered by a provider with a license to prescribe.

25. A home-care nurse is assessing a patient and family members from a cultural perspective. Which is **most** important for the nurse to do?
1. Recall experiences of caring for patients with a similar background.
2. Recognize beliefs common to the patient's ethnic group.
3. Interview the members of the patient's family.
4. Use the patient as the main source of data.

26. In which setting is it **most** essential for the nurse to assume multiple roles?
1. Rehabilitation facilities
2. Acute care hospitals
3. Rural communities
4. Urban centers

27. Which factor is essential to promote healthy lifestyles and behaviors within the community setting?
1. An entire family must be committed to making changes.
2. There must be resources available to support the desired changes.
3. The focus must be on the community as a whole, not on individuals.
4. A primary health-care provider's order is necessary before care can be provided.

28. A group of nurses is discussing various concerns about health care in the community setting in the United States. Which of the following should they include in the discussion because it has demonstrated a noticeable decline?
1. Public health organizations
2. At-risk patient groups
3. Cost of health care
4. Self-help groups

29. A community health nurse is to care for a patient who was just discharged from an acute care facility after receiving initial medical care for tuberculosis. The family recently immigrated to the United States from another country. Place the following interventions in the order in which they should be performed by the nurse.
1. Explore community resources that can help support the patient and family.
2. Perform an assessment of the patient and home environment.
3. Meet with the patient and family in their home.
4. Review the patient's medical record.
5. Identify patient and family needs.

Answer: ______________

30. Which statements reflect hospice care in the health-care delivery system? **Select all that apply.**
1. _____Patients must have less than half a year to live to receive services.
2. _____It assists families to care for their dying relatives at home.
3. _____Care is more expensive than in the acute care setting.
4. _____It provides mainly physical care to the dying person.
5. _____Hospice is a method of care rather than a location.

31. Identify the nursing interventions that reflect tertiary health-care services. **Select all that apply.**
1. _____Providing emotional support to family members after the death of a relative
2. _____Teaching a patient how to use a wheelchair after a stroke
3. _____Conducting a smoking cessation class
4. _____Administering an influenza vaccine
5. _____Changing a dressing after surgery

32. Which activities are examples of interventions associated with secondary health-care services? **Select all that apply.**
1. _____Conducting a cardiac risk assessment for middle-aged adults
2. _____Teaching a low-fat diet to a person with high cholesterol
3. _____Immunization of a child during the first year of life
4. _____Encouraging regular dental checkups
5. _____Monthly self-breast examinations

33. Which statements accurately reflect a concept about a healthy community? **Select all that apply.**
1. _____Health of a community is based on the sum of the health of its people.
2. _____The main focus in community health is on the health of each member of society.
3. _____A healthy community seeks to make community resources available to all members.
4. _____The focus of community health mainly is on healing the sick and preventing disease.
5. _____Promotion of health is one of the most important components of community health practice.

34. Which indictors are among the 10 leading health indicators identified by *Healthy People 2020*? **Select all that apply.**
1. _____Overweight and obesity
2. _____Substance abuse
3. _____Older adults
4. _____Diabetes
5. _____Vision

35. An older adult woman who has left-sided paralysis because of a brain attack is being cared for by a daughter in the home in which the daughter lives with her husband. The home-care nurse interviews each member of the family separately. Based on the significant information in each interview, which is the **most** important initial nursing intervention?
1. Be sensitive to the patient's cultural beliefs.
2. Arrange respite care for the patient's daughter.
3. Reinforce the daughter's responsibility to care for her mother.
4. Encourage the husband to help his wife with the care of his mother-in-law.

Interview With the Patient
"I am thankful that my daughter is caring for me. I took care of my parents and now it is my daughter's turn. Someday my daughter's children will be responsible for caring for her. I want to start acupuncture because I think it will help."

Interview With the Daughter
"Initially I took several months off from work to care for my mother. I know it is my responsibility to care for her but it is difficult because I work full time. She has me doing old-fashioned Asian remedies that take time and I don't even know if they will help."

Interview With the Daughter's Husband
"My mother-in-law came to live with us from Asia after her husband died. Since her recent discharge from the hospital my wife has been giving her heat and cold applications to promote harmony of yin and yang. It doesn't make any sense to me but my mother-in-law believes it works. I worry about my wife doing too much."

COMMUNITY-BASED NURSING: ANSWERS AND RATIONALES

1. 1. **A hospice program is an example of an agency that may provide or arrange for respite care in an inpatient setting or in the home. The caregiving role is physically and emotionally grueling, and family members may need relief from the caregiving role or a break to attend a family function or go on vacation.**
   2. Meals on Wheels does not provide respite care. It provides nutritious, low-cost meals for homebound people so that they can remain in their own homes.
   3. Ambulatory care centers do not provide respite care. Ambulatory care centers provide care for people with conditions that do not require hospitalization. Services may include diagnosis and treatment of disease and illness, as well as simple surgical procedures in which the patient returns home the same day.
   4. An alcohol treatment center does not provide respite care. It provides a specialized service in the care and treatment of individuals who abuse alcohol.

2. 1. Coordinating the efforts of the health-care team is an important responsibility of the nurse in all settings in which nurses work.
   2. Delivering skilled nursing care is an important responsibility of the nurse in all settings in which nurses work.
   3. Ensuring that patients receive healthy meals is an important responsibility of the nurse in all settings in which nurses work.
   4. **The hospital environment rarely requires modification because it is designed to provide for the safety needs of patients. However, in the home setting a home hazard assessment must be implemented to identify potential problems with walkways, stairways, floors, furniture, bathrooms, kitchens, electrical and fire protection, toxic substances, communication devices, and issues associated with medications and asepsis. Although the nurse may not be able to change a patient's living space and lifestyle, recommendations can be made that will minimize or eliminate risks.**

3. 1. The patient is the center of the health-care team in all settings.
   2. The nurse functions as an advocate for the patient in both the acute care and home-care settings. The role of advocate is important in all settings because in this role the nurse protects and supports patients' rights.
   3. The nurse is responsible for coordinating the efforts of the members of the health-care team in both the acute care and home-care settings.
   4. **Because of the shorter length of hospital stays, patients are being discharged before all teaching and counseling are completed. However, in the home-care setting, patients are provided with appropriate care until they are able to care for themselves.**

4. 1. Affirm means to state positively, to declare firmly, to ratify, and to assert. Exploring the nature and consequences of choices is not affirming.
   2. Mediate means to negotiate or intercede. Exploring the nature and consequences of choices is not mediating.
   3. **Inform means to give information, to enlighten, and to give knowledge. When working with families to explore the nature and consequences of their choices, the nurse can provide information so that people understand the ramifications of their choices. An informed decision is a decision based on an understanding of the facts and ramifications associated with the choice.**
   4. Interview means to meet and talk for the purpose of collecting information. Exploring the nature and consequences of choices is not interviewing. However, interviewing skills may be employed when the nurse explores with the patient the nature and consequences of choices.

5. 1. **As soon as contact with the patient is made, planning and teaching should begin so the patient is prepared to provide self-care in the home.**
   2. The nurse does not have to wait until the patient is admitted to the hospital to begin preparing for the patient's return to the community.

3. This is too late. The need for referrals to community agencies can be anticipated in most situations.
4. This is too late to prepare the patient for self-care in the community.

6. 1. This is not as important as an assessment presented in another option. The demographics of a community are only one component of a community assessment.
2. The members in the community are the primary source of data about the community and its needs. Just as the patient is the center of the health-care team when caring for an individual, the collective membership of a community is the center of the health-care team when caring for the health-care needs of a community.
3. This does not help to identify the needs of a community. After the needs of the community are identified, then the ability of the health-care system to deliver the necessary services is assessed.
4. This is not as important as an assessment presented in another option. Environmental data make up only one component of a community assessment.

7. 1. A middle school–aged child has to cope with the developmental conflict of Industry versus Inferiority. Tasks associated with this age such as deriving pleasure from accomplishments and developing a sense of competence can be facilitated in the home setting. Although a middle school–aged child will have to adjust to the need for long-term home health care, there are fewer crises occurring during the middle school years that impact on development than the number of crises occurring in a group in another option.
2. A preschool-aged child is dependent on a parent to provide for basic human needs and coping with the developmental conflict of Initiative versus Guilt. Tasks associated with this age, such as the development of confidence in ability and having direction and purpose, can be facilitated in the home setting. Although a preschool-aged child will have to adjust to the need for long-term home health care, there are fewer crises occurring during the preschool years that impact on development than the number of crises occurring in a group in another option.
3. Adolescents struggle with the developmental conflict of Identity versus Role Confusion. The adolescent generally will have the hardest time adjusting to the need for long-term home health care than any other stage of development. Adolescents experience multiple and complex physiological, psychological, and social developmental milestones. Adolescents want to be attractive to others, similar to their peers, and accepted within a group. It is common for adolescents to experience mood swings, make decisions without having all the facts, challenge authority, and assert the self. Being relatively isolated in the home for an extended period will pose serious stressors associated with adjustment, which can dramatically influence the outcome of the developmental tasks of adolescence.
4. The developmental conflict of Ego Integrity versus Despair challenges older adults to understand their worth and accept the approaching end of life. Although older adults will have the second-hardest time adjusting to the need for long-term home health care of the options offered, there are fewer crises occurring during the older adult years that impact development than the number of crises occurring in a group in another option.

8. 1. In the home setting, patients tend to have fewer health-care providers' orders and therefore nurses work more independently. In addition, the roles of the nurse in community-based practice today are expanding dramatically. In 1991, the American Nurses Association published *Nursing's Agenda for Health Care Reform*, which made recommendations for health-care reform. The major predictions influencing nurse accountability included: nurses will become community leaders; community-nursing centers will expand and focus on preventing disease and promoting health; and the center of health care will shift to the home setting. Nurses already work independently in such programs as community outreach, nursing centers, nurse-sponsored

wellness and health promotion programs, and independent practice. These roles require the nurse to utilize nursing theory and skills that are in the scope of the legal definition of nursing practice and do not require dependence on a primary health-care provider's orders.

2. Excellent communication skills are essential in both the acute care and community-based settings.
3. Teaching occurs in both the acute care and community-based settings. In addition, some patients may never be able to care for themselves.
4. Excellent technical skills are essential in both the acute care and community-based settings. Patients at home receive highly technical therapy such as hemodialysis, intravenous therapy, wound care, and ventilator support.

9. 1. This is not a safe place to keep medications. Children have natural curiosity, problem-solving abilities, and the agility to climb to a top shelf.

2. **A locked area is the safest place to store prescription as well as over-the-counter medications to prevent accidental ingestion by children.**
3. This is not a safe place to keep medications. Children have natural curiosity, problem-solving abilities, and the agility to climb up to a medicine cabinet.
4. This is not a safe place to keep medications. Children have natural curiosity and problem-solving abilities and could get to the back of a shelf in a refrigerator.

10. 1. The Occupational Therapist (OT) is not the most important member of the health-care team. An Occupational Therapist generally is not a member of the health-care team in an assisted-living residence. On occasion, a primary health-care provider may order occupational therapy, and either the resident will go to an Occupational Therapist to receive therapy or one will come to the resident and provide therapy.

2. Although Nurse Aides are the people who provide care related to activities of daily living needed by residents in an assisted-living residence, they are not as important as another member of the health-care team.
3. **The patient is always the center of the health-care team in every setting and is the most important member of the team.**
4. The nurse is not the most important health-care team member in an assisted-living facility. An assisted-living residence (i.e., apartment, villa, or condominium) provides limited assistance with activities of daily living, meal preparation, laundry services, transportation, and opportunities for socialization, not extensive nursing services.

11. 1. **Case management by the nurse in the home-care setting includes determining whether a patient is ready for discharge or requires a continuation of services. The nurse must document objectively the status of the patient to convince those making the decision (e.g., primary health-care provider, insurer, agency manager) that the patient requires a continuation of services. Nursing documentation supports the decision.**

2. Quality management activities are unrelated to whether a patient is to receive a continuation of services or is to be discharged from a home health-care program. Ongoing quality management programs are designed to monitor the quality of care being delivered and identify problem areas so that efforts can be employed to improve care.
3. Dissatisfaction with the services of a home health agency may influence whether or not the patient and/or family wants a continuation of services. However, satisfaction or dissatisfaction should not influence whether the patient still needs the services of the home health-care agency.
4. The primary health-care provider generally is not the only person making the decision of whether a patient is eligible for continuation of services or is ready for discharge from the home-care program. Agency managers and the insurer also may be involved in this decision. However, in the home-care setting a primary health-care provider's order is necessary to initiate home-care services as well as orders directing the nurse in the dependent functions of the nurse.

12. 1. Although it is important to have access to medical specialists, another option has priority. In addition, the availability of primary health-care providers, not specialists, is more essential because primary health care addresses health promotion, illness prevention, and entry into secondary health care (diagnosis and treatment of illness and disease).

2. Although individuals with health insurance have better access to health-care services, it is not essential to have health insurance to receive health care. People can pay privately or, if indigent, they can apply for various government and nonprofit-supported programs that provide basic care. In addition, hospital emergency departments, by law, cannot turn away patients who need emergency care.

3. For a healthy community, all members of the community must have access to health care. The health of a community depends on each member of the community having appropriate and comprehensive health care.

4. Public Health Nurses work for only the federal, state, or local governments implementing programs supported by taxes. These programs are only a small percentage of the multitude of programs and services that are designed to support community health.

13. 1. This is not the most efficient approach. This may be necessary if present resources are not available to meet the needs of the community.

2. The health needs of the members of the community are identified already. Further study at this time does not appear to be appropriate.

3. Designing educational approaches is not the most efficient approach. This may eventually be done after an action in another option is implemented first.

4. This is the most efficient initial approach to meeting the identified needs of the members of the community. The use of currently available resources is more efficient than the other options presented.

14. 1. The first and most important assessment made by the home-care nurse focuses on determining whether the patient's home environment is safe. Safety and security are basic needs identified by Maslow's Hierarchy of Needs.

2. Although it is often helpful when family members participate in a home-care patient's recovery, it is not necessary.

3. A patient's potential for self-care is not a criterion for receiving home-care services. Patients who have little or no potential for self-care receive home-care services.

4. Patients who are unable to participate in the plan of care because they are mentally, emotionally, or physically disabled are still eligible for home care.

15. 1. This scenario is not an example of an opinion survey. An opinion survey is designed to collect each individual person's perspective about the problem being studied. Results are tallied to identify the major concerns. Opinion surveys generally are questionnaires.

2. A forum is defined as an opportunity for open discussion. Inviting people from the community to share opinions and concerns about a particular issue for the purpose of collecting data is called a community forum.

3. This scenario is not an example of a demographic assessment. A demographic assessment is the quantitative study of the characteristics of a population. A demographic assessment might include information such as distribution of the population by gender, size, growth, density, and ethnicity.

4. This scenario is not an example of an observation of participants. Direct observation is a method of data collection that may be used to determine whether individuals follow a specific procedure or behave in an expected manner.

16. 1. Case management is a major role of the nurse in the home-care setting. The nurse engages in activities such as assessing, planning, coordinating nursing care and professional services, making referrals, monitoring medical progress, maintaining documentation, evaluating and monitoring outcomes, determining closure, and facilitating discharge of the patient after goal achievement.

2. Although discharge planning is a component of the role of the nurse in the home-care setting, it is not the role with the highest priority. Traditionally,

discharge planning was focused on moving a person from the hospital to the home. However, in the present health-care environment discharge planning is conducted when moving a patient from one level of care to another, which occurs in many settings.

3. Although family support is helpful, the patient's interest and motivation in achieving expected outcomes are the most important contributing factors to success.
4. The role of the nurse is to help the patient achieve expected outcomes that are within the patient's present value and belief systems. Although a patient might be healthier if other behaviors were adopted, it is difficult, and sometimes impossible, to change or modify a person's values and beliefs.

17. 1. Primary health-care providers' offices are the traditional primary care setting for ambulatory care. Patients go to primary health-care providers' offices for routine physicals and the diagnosis and treatment of routine illnesses or diseases. Follow-up visits to primary health-care providers are only one aspect of comprehensive health care.

2. Home-care agencies are responsible for coordinating and providing for a continuum of comprehensive health-care services after a patient is discharged from the hospital. Because of the decreased length of stay in the hospital setting, patients are being discharged sooner than ever before and are in need of home-care services.

3. Urgent visit centers are designed to diagnose and treat noncritical health problems, such as infections, minor injuries, and physical responses to disease or illness as well as primary care services.
4. Respite programs provide for short-stay, intermittent, inpatient, or day-care services to patients who generally are cared for at home. This service provides a rest period for family members who have the responsibility of sustained caregiving.

18. 1. Although the general health of members of a community is important, it is not the first information that the nurse should collect when assessing a community.

2. Acquiring core information about the people in the community is the first stage in assessing a community. Core characteristics about the members of a community include information such as vital statistics, values and beliefs, demographics, religious groups, and so on.

3. Although a community's physical environment (e.g., information such as whether it is rural, suburban, or urban, physical boundaries, density, size, types of lodgings, and incidence of crime) is important to know, it is not the first information that the nurse should collect when assessing a community.
4. Although it is important to know information such as agencies and services available, the accessibility to health-care services, sources of health information, transportation services, routine caseloads, and so on, it is not the first information that the nurse should collect when assessing a community.

19. 1. Families are not limited to individuals who are related by blood, marriage, adoption, or birth.

2. This is an example of a nuclear family and is only one example of a family structure.

3. A family is defined as a social group whose members are closely related by blood, marriage, or friendship. Today, family structure is diverse and includes types such as traditional nuclear families, single-parent families, blended families, cohabitating families, families with gay and lesbian members, families with foster children, and single people living alone but who are part of an extended family.

4. Family members remain connected by their relationships, not because they all live in the same household.

20. 1. Although this is a good idea, it is not the most important factor a home-care nurse can convey to a person caring for a family member in the home.

2. Although this might contribute to efficiency as well as gaining a feeling of control over the activities that must be accomplished, it is not the most important factor a home-care nurse can convey to a person caring for a family member in the home.
3. A daily journal of the patient's status is unnecessary when a patient is in stable condition. If the patient experiences an

acute episode, then a record of the patient's daily status could be helpful in monitoring progress or lack of progress.

4. Caregiver role strain experienced by a family member is a serious concern of home-care nurses. Caregivers often fail to address their own health needs because of the extraordinary burden of the caregiver role, which can jeopardize their own health and well-being. Caregivers should be encouraged to delegate responsibilities to other family members; get adequate sleep, rest, and nutritional intake; seek assistance from agencies that provide respite services; take time for leisure activities and a vacation; and join a caregiver support group.

21. 1. Critical care lies in the category of secondary, not tertiary, level of health-care services. The secondary level of health-care services is associated with acute care, complex diagnosis, treatment of disease and illness, and emergency care.

2. Long-term care lies in the category of tertiary level of health-care services. The tertiary level of health-care services is associated with rehabilitation, care of the dying, and long-term care.

3. Diagnostic care lies in the category of secondary, not tertiary, level of health-care services.

4. Preventive care lies in the category of primary, not tertiary, level of health-care services. Primary health-care services are concerned with promoting health and preventing disease.

22. 1. Hospice services are designed to assist patients who have less than 6 months to live and who have chosen to forego additional curative treatment for palliative care and support of quality of life. Hospice programs also provide support services to members of the patient's family as well as bereavement care for significant others after the death of the patient.

2. Although church outreach programs may be able to provide some support services, generally they are not able to provide the multiple services needed or to coordinate the continuum of comprehensive services that a person with functional deficits will require. Many church outreach programs generally serve as a source of information about services and programs available in the community, and they provide additional support that augments home-care services.

3. A home health-care agency is designed to coordinate the comprehensive services that a patient may need to recover from an illness that has caused functional deficits. This person may require help in areas such as assistance with activities of daily living, physical and occupational rehabilitation, direct nursing care, counseling, and so on.

4. Meals on Wheels provides for only the nutritional needs of a patient.

23. 1. This is not common to all medication containers. Only medications in liquid form should have drip-proof tops.

2. Most prescriptions filled for home use are in multidose containers.

3. Not all medications must be protected from the sun.

4. All prescriptions filled for home use are dispensed in containers with child-resistant tops, as required by law. If a person has a physical limitation, such as arthritis, that interferes with his or her ability to open a medication container, the person can request that a nonsafety top be provided. The pharmacy generally will document the request in its computer and may even require that a waiver be signed and witnessed for the record.

24. 1. The ability to provide some self-care is not necessary. In some instances, family members provide total care with no help from the patient.

2. A person does not have to have adequate financial resources to receive nursing services in the home. For example, Medicare, Medicaid, or private health-care insurance plans assume some of the costs of care provided in the home.

3. The presence of family members is not a requirement for home-care services. However, if it is unsafe for the patient to be home alone or unattended for long periods, the home may not be the most appropriate setting. In addition, patients who have no family support may rely on a friend, neighbor, or volunteers from a neighborhood outreach group to help in a supportive way.

4. **Health-care professionals who have prescriptive licenses (e.g., physicians, nurse practitioners, physician's assistants) must order home-care nursing services. An order from a provider with a prescriptive license is required if a home-care agency is to receive reimbursement from third-party sources (e.g., government, medical insurance plans). Orders written by these professionals direct the medical plan of care.**

25. 1. This denies the individuality of the patient. The nurse's experiential background may be limited and is influenced by personal views that may not be accurate.
2. Each patient is an individual, and generalizations should not be made based on a person's ethnic or cultural group. Generalizations often are based on stereotypes that are preconceived and untested beliefs about people based on their culture, race, and/or ethnic backgrounds.
3. Family members provide only their own views, which are not the most important when assessing variables that affect a patient from a cultural perspective.
4. **The patient is the center of the health-care team and is the most important source of information about his or her perspective.**

26. 1. Of the options presented, nurses working in a rehabilitation setting are less likely to assume multiple roles. Generally, nurses working in a rehabilitation setting have specific roles and responsibilities.
2. Of the options presented, nurses working in the acute care setting are less likely to assume multiple roles. Generally, nurses working in acute care settings have specific roles and responsibilities.
3. **Nurses working in rural communities wear many hats. The adage "wear many hats" refers to someone with many different roles and responsibilities. Rural refers to the country or the farm, where communities are less populated and are a great distance from primary health-care providers and health-care services. Because of the uneven distribution of health-care professionals and services in rural areas versus urban areas, nurses working in a rural area will assume many different roles and perform a variety of tasks.**
4. Of the options presented, nurses working in urban centers are less likely to assume multiple roles. Urban centers refer to cities with a population of more than 50,000 individuals, and they tend to have a concentration of specialized services where nurses have specific roles and responsibilities.

27. 1. Each individual person is responsible for his or her own health-seeking actions and behavior. It is ideal if all members of a family are interested and motivated to promote a healthy lifestyle; however, not all members of a family are committed to this value.
2. **Resources that support health promotion, health protection, and preventive health services are essential if one expects members of the community to engage in healthy lifestyles and behaviors. Resources, such as availability of health professionals, sites for primary health prevention programs for meetings and provision of services, consumables in the form of equipment and medications (e.g., immunizations), and so on, must be available to promote and support health.**
3. Although programs are designed to meet the needs of groups in a community, each individual must be reached and influenced when promoting healthy lifestyles and behaviors.
4. Education is the key in relation to recognizing and understanding the importance of behaviors that support a healthy lifestyle. Educational intervention is an independent function of the nurse and does not require a primary health-care provider's order.

28. 1. **Public health agencies established at the federal, state, and local levels to safeguard and improve the physical, mental, and social well-being of an entire community are on the decline. In an effort to reduce the escalating rise in the budgets of public health agencies, programs and services have been reduced or terminated.**
2. The number of patient groups at risk is increasing, not declining; for example, groups such as older adults, the homeless,

the uninsured, people living below the poverty level, single-parent families, and immigrants.

3. The cost of health care in the United States is dramatically increasing, not declining. In 2011 17.9% of the gross domestic product was spent on health-care costs. It is predicted that by 2021 health-care costs will be 19.9% of the gross domestic product and they will be 26% to 30% by 2040.
4. The number of self-help groups is increasing, not declining. More than 500 self-help groups represent almost all the major health problems, life events, or crises. The National Self-Help Clearinghouse provides information about existing groups and guidelines on how to begin a new group. Consumer access to the World Wide Web and the Internet has disseminated information about self-help groups.

29. **4. Before meeting with the patient and family the nurse should obtain as much information about the patient as possible.**

3. An assessment of the home environment can be performed only in the home. The patient's family members should be included when feasible because they may provide emotional support and/or be involved with physical care of the patient.

2. A health history and physical assessment of the patient should be performed by the community health nurse. The information on the patient's clinical record may not reflect the patient's current status. The home must be assessed to ensure that it is a safe environment for the patient and that care can be delivered adequately to meet the patient's needs.

5. The nurse, in conjunction with the patient (and family members when appropriate), must identify present needs. Once this is accomplished then goals and objectives can be identified and a plan of care formulated.

1. Once a plan of care is formulated then the nurse, in conjunction with the patient (and family members when appropriate), can identify community resources that may assist them in attaining the goals and objectives of the plan of care.

30. **1. To be eligible for hospice services, an individual must be diagnosed as having less than 6 months to live. It is a service to support patients and their families through the process of dying.**

2. Most hospice care is delivered in patients' homes supported by a team of health-care providers and volunteers. However, there are inpatient hospice programs, palliative care units in hospitals, and residential hospice settings.

3. The home is a less expensive setting than other health-care settings because family members provide most of the care supported by a team of professionals, nonprofessionals, and volunteers.

4. Hospice services include not only palliative physical care and support of quality of life for the terminally ill patient but also emotional support to patients and family members. In addition, they include services that assist family members with bereavement and adjustment after the death of the patient.

5. Hospice is not a location but a concept. It provides supportive, palliative services that focus on managing pain, treatment of symptoms, and helping patients maintain their quality of life so they can live the remainder of their lives to the fullest.

31. **1. Providing bereavement services is an example of a tertiary health-care service. Tertiary care is associated with rehabilitation, long-term care, and care of the dying. Health-care services, which describe the scope of services and settings where health care is provided, include primary, secondary, and tertiary levels. The levels of health-care services should not be confused with levels of prevention.**

2. Teaching a patient how to use a wheelchair after a stroke is an example of a tertiary health-care service. Tertiary services provide care related to rehabilitation.

3. A smoking cessation class is an example of a service provided on the primary, not tertiary, level of health-care services. Primary health care is associated with illness prevention, health promotion, environmental protection, and health education.

4. Immunizations are an example of primary, not tertiary, health-care services. Primary health care is concerned with promoting health, preventing disease, environmental protection, and health education.
5. Changing a dressing after surgery is care associated with the secondary, not tertiary, level of health-care services. Secondary health care is associated with acute care, complex diagnosis and treatment of disease and illness, and emergency care.

32. 1. This is a primary, not secondary, health-care service. Risk assessments for specific diseases are included in primary health-care services. Primary health-care services are concerned with generalized health promotion and specific protection against disease.
2. A low-fat diet generally is part of a medical management program for a person who is overweight or who has high cholesterol. This is a tertiary, not secondary, health-care service. Tertiary health-care services are associated with attempts to reduce the extent and severity of a health problem in an effort to limit disability as well as restore and maintain function.
3. Administering an immunization is a primary, not secondary, health-care service. Primary health-care services include protecting people from disease.
4. Encouraging regular dental checkups is a secondary health-care service that is associated with early detection of disease and prompt intervention.
5. Monthly self-breast examinations are associated with secondary health-care services because they are concerned with detection of breast cancer.

33. 1. This statement does not accurately reflect a concept about a healthy community. A healthy community seeks to provide infrastructure, resources, and activities that support a healthy community and is not just reflective of the health of its members.
2. This is not an accurate statement. Community health focuses on families, groups, and the community, not just individuals.
3. A healthy community is concerned about all members of the community and works to ensure that all members have access to all of the system's resources.
4. This statement focuses on illness and is too limited in relation to community health.
5. Health promotion has taken on new meaning as consumers take more responsibility for their health status. Teaching about promoting health is a more positive perspective than teaching about preventing illness, which is a negative perspective.

34. 1. Overweight and obesity is one of the 10 leading health indicators identified by *Healthy People 2020*. The other nine topics are physical activity, substance abuse, tobacco use, responsible sexual behavior, mental health, injury and violence, environmental quality, immunization, and access to health care.
2. Substance abuse is one of the 10 leading health indicators identified by *Healthy People 2020*. The other nine topics are physical activity, overweight and obesity, tobacco use, responsible sexual behavior, mental health, injury and violence, environmental quality, immunization, and access to health care.
3. Older adults is not one of the 10 leading health indicators, but it is one of the 42 topic areas.
4. Diabetes is not one of the 10 leading health indicators, but it is one of the 42 topic areas.
5. Vision is not one of the 10 leading health indicators, but it is one of the 42 topic areas.

35. 1. Beliefs and values usually are held long term and are engrained within one's view of self. It is essential that nurses respect a patient's beliefs and values, particularly for nontraditional healing practices as long as they are not harmful to the patient. Demonstrating respect and a nonjudgmental attitude will help promote a trusting nurse-patient relationship.
2. Arranging respite care for the daughter is premature at this time. This may eventually become necessary.
3. This is an inappropriate intervention by the nurse. Only the daughter can come to the conclusion that it is her responsibility to care for her mother.
4. This is not the priority. This intervention may be done after a discussion with the patient, daughter, and husband.

3 Psychosociocultural Nursing Care

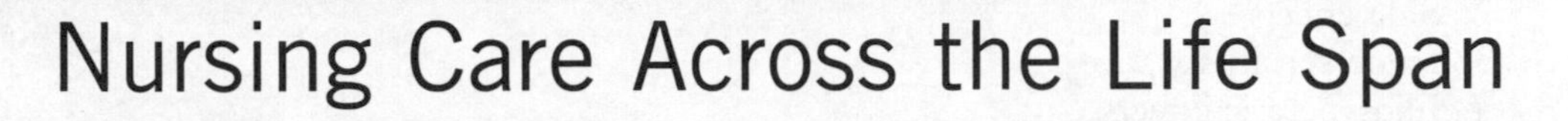

Nursing Care Across the Life Span

KEYWORDS

The following words include nursing/medical terminology, concepts, principles, and information relevant to content specifically addressed in the chapter or associated with topics presented in it. English dictionaries, nursing textbooks, and medical dictionaries, such as *Taber's Cyclopedic Medical Dictionary,* are resources that can be used to expand your knowledge and understanding of these words and related information.

Adolescent (teenager)
Agism
Attachment, bonding
Brazelton, Berry—Neonatal Behavioral Assessment Scale
Cephalocaudal
Congenital anomalies
Critical time
Developmental:
- Milestones
- Stressor
- Task

Egocentrism
Erikson, Erik—Theory of Personality Development
Failure to thrive
Fetus
Fowler, James—Theory of Faith Development
Freud, Sigmund—Psychoanalytical Theory
Genetics
Havighurst, Robert—Developmental Task Theory of Development
Infancy, infant, neonate, newborn
Kohlberg, Lawrence—Theory of Moral Development
Life cycle
Life events
Low birth weight
Maslow, Abraham—Hierarchy of Basic Human Needs
Menarche
Menopause
Middle adulthood
Midlife crisis
Moral reasoning
Older adult
Organogenesis
Physique
Piaget, Jean—Cognitive Development Theory
Premenopausal, postmenopausal
Preschool-aged child
Preterm
Proximodistal
Psychosocial development
Puberty
Regression
Retirement
Role reversal
Sandwich generation
School-aged child
Senescence
Sibling rivalry
Teratogenic
Toddler
Young adulthood

NURSING CARE ACROSS THE LIFE SPAN: QUESTIONS

1. A nurse is administering medication to an older adult. For which response to medication that occurs **most** frequently in older adults should the nurse assess the patient?
   1. Toxicity
   2. Side effects
   3. Hypersensitivity
   4. Idiosyncratic effects

2. A nurse in a clinic is caring for patients in a variety of age groups. Which age group should the nurse anticipate will have the greatest potential to demonstrate regression when ill?
   1. Infants
   2. Toddlers
   3. Adolescents
   4. Young adults

3. When the nurse assesses an adult patient, which patient behavior may indicate an unresolved developmental task of infancy?
   1. Avoiding assistance from others
   2. Rationalizing unacceptable behaviors
   3. Being overly concerned about cleanliness
   4. Apologizing constantly for small mistakes

4. Which patient should the nurse identify is at the **greatest** risk when taking a drug that has a high teratogenic potential?
   1. Older adult man
   2. Pregnant woman
   3. Four-year-old child
   4. One-month-old infant

5. A nurse in the emergency department is assessing patients of various ages. Which age group should the nurse anticipate will have the **greatest** individual differences in appearance and behavior?
   1. Children
   2. Adolescents
   3. Older adults
   4. Middle-aged adults

6. A 70-year-old patient tells the nurse about experiencing problems with sleep and requests sleeping medication. Which concept associated with drug therapy and quality of sleep is important for the nurse to explain when providing nursing care for this patient?
   1. Sedatives are not well tolerated by older adults.
   2. Antianxiety drugs are the least helpful to support sleep.
   3. Effectiveness of hypnotics increases with prolonged use.
   4. Melatonin is the drug of choice for long-term use in sleep disorders.

7. Which concept is reflective of Erik Erikson's Theory of Personality Development?
   1. Defense mechanisms help people to cope with anxiety.
   2. Moral maturity is a central theme in all stages of development.
   3. Achievement of developmental goals is affected by the social environment.
   4. Two continual processes, assimilation and accommodation, stimulate intellectual growth.

8. A nurse in the clinic is monitoring patients for iron deficiency anemia. Which group of individuals should the nurse anticipate to be at the **greatest** risk?
   1. Postmenopausal women
   2. Older adults
   3. Teenagers
   4. Infants

9. Which group of individuals should the nurse anticipate is at the **greatest** risk for constipation?
   1. Inactive school-aged children
   2. Middle-aged adults
   3. Older-aged adults
   4. Bottle-fed infants

10. A parent tells the nurse in the well-child clinic that the 2-year-old is trying to eat with a spoon and is making a mess. Which should the nurse encourage the parent to do?
    1. Praise and encourage the child while eating.
    2. Provide finger foods until the child is older.
    3. Feed the child along with the child's attempts at eating.
    4. Take the spoon and feed the child until the child is more capable.

11. One of the participants attending a parenting seminar asks the nurse teaching the class, "What is the leading cause of death during the first year of life?" Besides exploring the person's concerns, what should the nurse respond?
    1. Sudden infant death syndrome
    2. Congenital malformations
    3. Unintentional injuries
    4. Short gestation

12. Which individual does the nurse anticipate has the **greatest** risk for problems with regulating body temperature?
    1. Toddler
    2. Teenager
    3. Older adult
    4. School-aged child

13. A pediatric nurse is caring for children of a variety of ages. Which group should the nurse anticipate will have the **most** problems sleeping as a result of multiple complex developmental factors?
    1. Infants
    2. Toddlers
    3. Adolescents
    4. Preschoolers

14. Which is a person referring to when during an interview the person says, "I am a member of the *sandwich generation*"?
    1. Cares for children and aging parents at the same time
    2. Has reversed roles between parents and self
    3. Assists own parents and spouse's parents
    4. Has both older and younger siblings

15. A nurse is planning a teaching session for an older adult about a prescribed medication regimen. Which is a major concern about older adults that the nurse should consider?
    1. They experience an increase in absorption of drugs from the gastrointestinal tract.
    2. They are less motivated to follow a prescribed drug regimen.
    3. They often use alcohol to cope with the stressors of aging.
    4. They have a decreased risk for adverse reactions to drugs.

16. A nurse is caring for several children on a pediatric unit. Children in which age group should the nurse expect will be **most** unstable and challenging with regard to the development of a personal identity?
    1. Toddlerhood
    2. Adolescence
    3. Childhood
    4. Infancy

17. A nurse in the operating room cares for patients of a variety of ages. Which individual should the nurse anticipate will have the **greatest** risk for complications during surgery?
    1. Middle-aged adult
    2. Pregnant woman
    3. Adolescent
    4. Infant

18. Which word describes the process of growth and development?
    1. Fast
    2. Simple
    3. Limiting
    4. Individual

19. A hospice nurse is providing emotional support for eight young children of a dying mother. At which age do children first recognize that death is irreversible, universal, and natural?
    1. 9 years of age
    2. 6 years of age
    3. 15 years of age
    4. 12 years of age

20. A school nurse is teaching a class of adolescents about nutrition. Which age group should the nurse identify as having the **highest** energy expenditure and nutrient requirements?
    1. End of the life cycle
    2. Middle adult years
    3. Early adult years
    4. First year of life

21. A nurse determines that according to Erikson, establishing relationships based on commitment mainly occurs in which stage of psychosocial development?
    1. Middle-aged adulthood
    2. Young adulthood
    3. Adolescence
    4. Infancy

22. Which age group should the nurse identify as being reflected in the following statement? "More time is spent in bed but less time is spent asleep."
    1. Two-year-olds
    2. Forty-year-olds
    3. Seventy-year-olds
    4. Fourteen-year-olds

23. A nurse is teaching a parenting class at a local community health center. Which common stressor associated with the developmental stage of early childhood (1 to 3 years) should the nurse include?
    1. Accepting limited dietary choices
    2. Adjusting to a change in physique
    3. Responding to life-threatening illness
    4. Resolving conflicts associated with independence

24. A nurse is providing dietary teaching to a group of adolescents recently diagnosed with diabetes mellitus. Which factor should the nurse consider that frequently influences food choices by adolescents?
1. Taste
2. Routine
3. Pressure
4. Preference

25. Which common physiological changes associated with aging should the nurse assess for in an older adult? **Select all that apply.**
1. _____Increase in sebaceous gland activity
2. _____Deterioration of joint cartilage
3. _____Loss of social support system
4. _____Decreased hearing acuity
5. _____Increased need for sleep

26. A nurse is facilitating a mothers' class, and the women begin discussing experiences that reflect the intellectual development of their children. Each woman describes a situation that reflects one of the stages of Jean Piaget's theory about logical thinking. Place the situations described in order beginning with the sensorimotor stage and ending with formal operations.
1. "My son touched the radiator and got burned. He'll never do that again."
2. "My son is learning math and is getting 100s on his tests. He is so smart."
3. "My daughter is on the debating team in school. We go to interschool meets."
4. "My daughter asked an obese lady if she had a baby in her stomach. I was so embarrassed."

Answer: ____________________

27. A nurse identifies that an older adult has successfully resolved the developmental conflict associated with aging. Which of the person's abilities **most** support this conclusion? **Select all that apply.**
1. _____Accepting social isolation
2. _____Reminiscing about past life events
3. _____Managing the change in social roles
4. _____Associating with members of every age group
5. _____Increasing the number of meaningful relationships

28. An older adult is admitted to the intensive care unit. For which common adaptations to sensory overload should the nurse monitor the patient? **Select all that apply.**
1. _____Tachycardia
2. _____Drowsiness
3. _____Confusion
4. _____Irritability
5. _____Dementia

29. A nurse identifies which words as being **unrelated** to principles of growth and development? **Select all that apply.**
1. _____Unpredictable
2. _____Sequential
3. _____Integrated
4. _____Simple
5. _____Static

30. A nurse identifies that a patient in middle adulthood is experiencing a developmental crisis. Which of the person's behaviors support this conclusion? **Select all that apply.**
1. _____Unable to mentor children in the next generation
2. _____Difficulty in developing peer relationships
3. _____Inability to achieve feelings of success
4. _____Incapable of delaying satisfaction
5. _____Failure to face eventual death

31. A school nurse is assessing several school-aged children between the ages of 6 and 12 years. Which assessment of a child requires a further assessment?
1. 7-year-old boy
2. 9-year-old girl
3. 11-year-old boy
4. 12-year-old girl

7-Year-Old Boy Grew 1 inch in the last year Gained 15 pounds in the last year
9-Year-Old Girl Concerned about achieving acceptable grades in school Identifies with other girls in her grade
11-Year-Old Boy Appears clumsy Is tall and thin
12-Year-Old Girl Concerned about her physical appearance Interested in boys

32. A nurse is caring for a variety of individuals across the life span. Which age groups generally demonstrate an inefficiency of adaptation? **Select all that apply.**
1. _____More than 60 years
2. _____40 to 60 years
3. _____12 to 19 years
4. _____3 to 11 years
5. _____0 to 1 year

33. A nurse identifies that an adult has an unresolved developmental conflict associated with adolescence. Which behaviors support this conclusion? **Select all that apply.**
1. _____Being overly concerned about following daily routines
2. _____Requiring excessive attention from others
3. _____Relying on oneself rather than others
4. _____Failing to verbalize a sense of self
5. _____Lacking goals in life

34. Which family members comments about an older adult member of the family demonstrates agism? **Select all that apply.**
1. _____"She has outlived her usefulness."
2. _____"She is elderly but she is so cute."
3. _____"She reads the newspaper with difficulty."
4. _____"He reminisces about his past work experience."
5. _____"He is most happy when working in his home workshop."

35. A nurse is assessing a 4-year-old child's growth and development. Which activities should the nurse expect the child to be capable of performing? **Select all that apply.**
1. _____Dresses self
2. _____Uses toy tools
3. _____Hops on one foot
4. _____Rides a two-wheel bicycle
5. _____Swims using the freestyle stroke

NURSING CARE ACROSS THE LIFE SPAN: ANSWERS AND RATIONALES

1. **1. This is a serious concern because of a decrease in efficiency of hepatic metabolism and renal excretion of drugs in older adults; as a result, accumulation of the drug occurs, resulting in toxicity.**
2. Although side effects are a concern in older adults, another option is a greater concern.
3. Although hypersensitivity is a concern in older adults, another option is a greater concern.
4. Although idiosyncratic effects are a concern in older adults, another option is a greater concern.

2. 1. Infants already demonstrate behavior on the most basic level.
2. Toddlers are less able to understand and interpret what is happening to them when ill; therefore, they commonly regress to a previous level of development in an attempt to reduce anxiety.
3. Adolescents generally want to behave in an adult manner and therefore demonstrate a controlled behavioral response to illness.
4. Although some young adults may regress to an earlier level of development as a coping strategy, regression commonly is not used as a defense mechanism when coping with illness.

3. **1. People who avoid help from others and who would rather do things themselves generally have not completely resolved the developmental task of Trust versus Mistrust during infancy.**
2. Rationalizing unacceptable behaviors is a defense mechanism, not an indication of an unresolved developmental task of infancy. Rationalization is used to justify in some socially acceptable way ideas, feelings, or behavior through explanations that appear to be logical.
3. This behavior relates more to the Anal Stage of Freud's Psychosexual Theory of Development. Freud believed that when toilet training is approached in a rigid and demanding manner, a child develops into an adult who is overly concerned with orderliness and cleanliness.
4. This may indicate an unresolved conflict of Autonomy versus Shame and Doubt associated with the 18-month- to 3-year-old age group. One of the developmental tasks of this age group is learning right from wrong. When parents are overly critical and controlling, a child may be overly self-judgmental and become an adult who feels the need to apologize for small mistakes constantly.

4. 1. An older adult man is not at risk when receiving a medication that has a teratogenic effect.
2. A pregnant woman is at risk. Teratogenic refers to a substance that can cross the placental barrier and interfere with growth and development of the fetus.
3. A 4-year-old child is not at risk when receiving a medication that has a teratogenic effect.
4. A newborn is not at risk when receiving a medication that has a teratogenic effect.

5. 1. School-aged children (6 to 12 years) tend to have fewer differences in appearance and behavior from their peers. These children begin to be involved with formalized groups where conformity is expected.
2. Although adolescents (12 to 20 years) may be viewed as different from the norms of their parents, they are similar to their peers. In their search for self-identity, adolescents experience role confusion. To control anxiety with role confusion, they are attracted to and conform to peer groups, which provide a sense of security.
3. Although there is diversity in the older adult group (65 years or older) individuals have to adjust to common experiences such as physical decline, retirement, multiple losses, and changes in social roles. Older adults commonly seek out people of the same age to share similar interests and find status among their peers.
4. Middle-aged adults (40 to 60 years) are in a time of transition between young adulthood and older adulthood. Therefore, individuals in this group, more so than in any other age group, have the greatest individual differences

in appearance and behavior as they span the norms seen in young adulthood, middle adulthood, and older adulthood.

6. **1. Sedatives are not well tolerated by older adults because a decrease in the metabolism and excretion of the drug can result in toxicity. In addition, older adults may experience idiosyncratic (e.g., unexpected or opposite) effects.**
2. Antianxiety drugs depress the central nervous system and therefore are helpful in supporting sleep.
3. The effectiveness of hypnotics decreases, not increases, with prolonged use. They should be used only as a short-term intervention because tolerance and rebound insomnia occur in approximately four weeks.
4. Although melatonin demonstrates promise as a drug to support sleep, it is not the drug of choice because its safety and efficacy are not yet established.

7. 1. Sigmund Freud, not Erik Erikson, identified that defense mechanisms are used to reduce anxiety by preventing conscious awareness of threatening thoughts or feelings.
2. Lawrence Kohlberg, not Erik Erikson, established a framework for understanding the development of moral maturity, which is the ability to recognize independently what is right and what is wrong.
3. Erik Erikson expanded on Freud's Theory of Personality Development by giving equal emphasis to the influence of a person's social and cultural environment. He stressed that psychosocial development depends on an interactive process between the physical and emotional variables during a person's life at eight distinct stages. Each stage requires resolution of a developmental conflict that has opposite outcomes and that requires interaction within the self and with others in the environment.
4. Assimilation and accommodation of new information necessary to stimulate intellectual growth comprise a concept basic to Jean Piaget's Theory of Cognitive Development, not Erikson's Theory of Personality Development. Assimilation involves the process of organizing new information into one's present body of knowledge, and accommodation involves rearranging and restructuring thought processes to deal with the imbalance caused by new information and thereby increase understanding.

8. 1. Cessation of estrogen and progesterone production during menopause does not contribute to iron deficiency anemia.
2. Although older adults are at risk for iron deficiency anemia because of decreased intake and less efficient absorption of nutrients, they are not at as high a risk as an age group in another option.
3. Although teenagers are at risk for iron deficiency anemia because of rapid growth and diets high in fat and low in vitamins, they are not at as high a risk as an age group in another option.
4. Infants are at the highest risk for iron deficiency anemia because of the increased physiological demand for blood production during growth, inadequate solid food intake after 6 months of age, and formula not fortified with iron. In addition, premature or multiple-birth infants are at special risk because of inadequate stores of iron during the end of fetal development.

9. 1. Although inactivity may promote constipation, there are no physiological changes in school-aged children that will compound the risk for constipation.
2. Although middle-aged adults experience slower gastrointestinal motility than when they were younger, they are not at as great a risk for constipation as an age group in another option.
3. Older adults are at the greatest risk for constipation because of decreases in activity levels, in intake of high-fiber foods, in peristalsis, in digestive enzymes, and in fluid intake.
4. Constipation in infants is uncommon except when they are weaned from formula to cow's milk or when their diet is mismanaged.

10. **1. From 18 months to 3 years of age (Autonomy versus Shame and Doubt), the child strives for independence. Attempts to self-feed should be encouraged and enthusiastically praised even though the child may make a mess. They allow the child to practice**

and perfect new skills, help to develop fine motor skills, and support control of the self and the environment.

2. Although finger foods help to avoid a mess during mealtime, the child must learn how to use utensils when eating. This intervention interferes with the achievement of the task associated with this age group.
3. This should be avoided. When children are made to feel that the job they are doing is not good enough, it conveys a sense of shame and doubt and will make them feel inadequate.
4. This is discouraging to the child and may precipitate feelings of inadequacy, shame, and doubt. When caregivers always do what children should be learning, children are not permitted to learn for themselves.

11. 1. The most recent statistics from the National Center for Health Statistics indicate that sudden infant death syndrome (SIDS) is ranked as the third leading cause of all infant deaths.

2. The most recent statistics from the National Center for Health Statistics indicate that congenital malformations are ranked first as the leading cause of all infant deaths.

3. The most recent statistics from the National Center for Health Statistics indicate that unintentional injuries are ranked as the fifth leading cause of all infant deaths. Maternal complications associated with pregnancy are ranked as the fourth leading cause of all infant deaths.
4. The most recent statistics from the National Center for Health Statistics indicate that short gestation and low birth weight are ranked as the second leading cause of all infant deaths.

12. 1. Toddlers generally are able to regulate body temperature as long as they are basically healthy.

2. Adolescents generally are able to regulate body temperature as long as there are no coexisting health problems.

3. Regulation of body temperature depends on the ability to dilate or constrict blood vessels and control the activity of sweat glands. In the older adult, the production of sweat glands decreases, reducing a person's ability to perspire and resulting in risk for heat exhaustion; there are decreased amounts of muscle mass and subcutaneous fat, which lead to increased susceptibility to cold; there are inefficient vasoconstriction in response to cold and inefficient vasodilation in response to heat; and there is a diminished ability to shiver.

4. School-aged children generally are able to regulate temperature as long as there are no other underlying medical conditions.

13. 1. Infants initially sleep 17 to 20 hours a day and by the end of the first year are sleeping 12 to 16 hours a day. Frequent awakening for feeding is expected and is not a sleep problem for the infant.

2. Toddlers (18 months to 3 years) generally sleep 12 to 15 hours a day with one or two naps. Toddlers occasionally will awaken during the night because of teething pains, illness, separation anxiety, and loneliness; awakening during the night is not unusual in the toddler. If caregivers establish regular bedtime routines and provide emotional comfort, sleep problems are minimal during this age group.

3. Adolescents (12 to 20 years) have more multiple and complex physiological (e.g., puberty), psychological (e.g., self-identity and independence issues), and social (e.g., peer pressure, altered roles, and maturing relationships) milestones than any other stage of development. Anxiety associated with all of these stressors contributes to altered sleep patterns and sleep deprivation. Adolescents generally need 8 to 10 hours of sleep a day; however, adolescents' sleep needs vary widely.

4. Preschoolers (3 to 5 years) have well-established sleep-wake cycles, they sleep 10 to 12 hours a day, and daytime napping decreases. Dreams and nightmares, which can awaken the child, are common but are not considered abnormal. Establishing consistent rituals that include quiet time helps to minimize nighttime awakening.

14. 1. When middle-aged adults are caring for their children and their aging, dependent parents at the same time, they are referred to as the sandwich generation. Their parents and children represent the bread, and they are the meat in between.

2. Role reversal is not a definition of the sandwich generation.
3. Assisting both sets of parents is not a definition of the sandwich generation.
4. Being a middle child between older and younger siblings is not the definition of the sandwich generation.

15. 1. Older adults experience decreased, not increased, absorption of drugs from the gastrointestinal tract.
2. The literature documents that older adults are at high risk for nonadherence to a medication regimen because of its complexity. The larger the number of medications and the larger the number of doses per day, the higher the risk of nonadherence. One study indicated that the adherence rate was 87% for daily dosing, 81% for doses twice a day, 77% for doses three times a day, and 39% for doses four times a day. Other reasons for not fully adhering to a drug regimen include inconvenience, side effects, financial limitations, and/or perceived ineffectiveness of the drugs.
3. Although approximately 10% to 15% of older adults have some problem with alcohol use late in life, the literature supports the fact that there is a decrease, not increase, in the incidence of alcoholism with the aged.
4. Older adults have an increased, not decreased, risk for adverse reactions to drugs. Adverse effects are any effects that are not therapeutic. Adverse effects can be side effects that are minor and tolerable or serious, requiring discontinuation of the drug.

16. 1. Although toddlers (18 months to 3 years; early childhood—Autonomy versus Shame and Doubt) experience a number of developmental milestones, toddlerhood is not as unstable or complex as another stage of development. Toddlers explore and test the environment, develop independence, and have a beginning ability to control the self.
2. Adolescents (12 to 20 years—Identity versus Role Confusion) have more multiple and complex physiological (e.g., puberty), psychological (e.g., self-identity and independence), and social (e.g., peer pressure, altered roles, and maturing relationships) milestones than any other stage of development. The multiplicity of these stressors can have a major impact on the development of the adolescent's personal identity and sense of self.
3. Although children in early childhood or toddlerhood (18 months to 3 years—Autonomy versus Shame and Doubt) and late childhood (3 to 6 years—Initiative versus Guilt) experience a number of developmental milestones, they are not as unstable or complex as another age group. The main tasks of childhood are achievement of self-control, initiation of one's own activities, and development of purpose and competence.
4. Although infants (birth to 18 months—Trust versus Mistrust) experience a number of developmental milestones, their development is not as unstable or complex as that of another age group. The main tasks of infancy are to adjust to living in and responding to the environment and the development of trust.

17. 1. Middle-aged adults usually are safe candidates for surgery.
2. Although a pregnant woman has unique needs during surgery, as long as the mother's cardiovascular and fluid and electrolyte statuses are maintained, the fetus is supported and safe.
3. Although the adolescent has needs related to body image and separation from friends, the physiological risk of surgery is not increased.
4. Infants are at risk for fluid volume depletion because of a small blood volume and limited fluid reserves. In addition, immature liver and kidneys affect the ability to metabolize and eliminate drugs, an undeveloped immune system increases the risk of infection, and immature temperature regulating mechanisms increase the risk of hyperthermia and hypothermia.

18. 1. Some stages are faster and some are slower, depending on the person and the developmental level.
2. The growth and development process is complex and influenced by many different factors.
3. Just the opposite is true; the growth and development process helps people to extend themselves to be the most that they can be.

4. **Although people follow a general pattern, they do not grow and develop at exactly the same rate or extent.**

19. 1. **A 9-year-old child has a more realistic understanding of death than a younger child and recognizes that death is universal, irreversible, and natural. A 9-year-old child has a beginning knowledge of his or her own mortality and may fear death.**
2. A 6-year-old child is developing an understanding of the differences among the concepts of past, present, and future. A 6-year-old child believes that death is temporary, can be caused by bad thoughts, and may be a punishment and that magic can make the dead person alive.
3. Recognizing that death is irreversible, universal, and natural occurs at an earlier age than 15 years.
4. Recognizing that death is irreversible, universal, and natural occurs at an earlier age than 12 years.

20. 1. Older adults experience decreases in basal metabolic rate, lean body mass, and physical activity that contribute to a decrease in caloric needs.
2. During the middle adult years, energy expenditure decreases and nutritional needs stabilize. People in other age groups have greater needs for nutrients to meet physiological demands than do those in the middle adult years.
3. Although young adults tend to be active and require nutrients adequate to meet high energy expenditure, physical growth slows and the basal metabolic rate begins to stabilize, so they require fewer calories than do other age groups.
4. **During the first year of life, nutritional needs per unit of body weight are the greatest in comparison to any other time during the life span. Birth weight generally doubles in 4 to 6 months and triples by the end of the first year.**

21. 1. Middle-aged adults (25 to 45 years—Generativity versus Stagnation) strive to fulfill life goals associated with family, career, and society, as well as to give to and care for others.
2. **Young adults (18 to 25 years—Intimacy versus Isolation) strive to establish mature relationships, commit to suitable partners, and develop social and work roles acceptable to society. Unsuccessful resolution results in self-absorption, egocentricity, and emotional isolation.**
3. Adolescents (12 to 20 years—Identity versus Role Confusion) strive to make the transition from childhood to adulthood with a sense of personal self.
4. Infants (newborn to 18 months—Trust versus Mistrust) strive to have their needs met through interacting with others. When their needs are consistently met they develop a sense of trust in their caregivers.

22. 1. Toddlers are active once awake and rarely spend much time in bed when not sleeping. Toddlers sleep 12 to 14 hours a day, including one or two daytime naps.
2. Middle-aged adults sleep 6 to 8 hours a day. Although middle-aged adults spend more time in bed awake than when they were younger, they spend less time in bed awake than an age group in another option.
3. **Older adults still need 7 to 9 hours of sleep daily but often receive less because of difficulty falling asleep and more frequent awakening. They often go to bed earlier in an effort to get more sleep and end up spending more time in bed awake. Sleeping difficulties are attributed to a decrease in melatonin, less deep sleep, a decrease in exercise, more naps, movement disorders, sleep apnea, and medical and psychological problems.**
4. Adolescents sleep 8 to 10 hours a day. Adolescents generally have high activity levels and stay up late. It may seem as though adolescents are always sleeping because they sleep later in the morning, but generally they go to bed much later at night.

23. 1. This might be required of an older adult who is learning to adjust to a therapeutic diet. More often people in the older age group need to adapt to the stress of a declining ability to ingest, digest, and/or absorb particular food.
2. This is an expected developmental task of adolescence, not early childhood. Many bodily changes occur in this transitional period, such as a growth spurt and sexual maturity.
3. This is not an expected developmental stressor of this age group. Only a small

percentage of the population of 18-month-old to 3-year-old children faces the challenge of a life-threatening illness.

4. **During early childhood, the child gains independence through learning right from wrong. Independence occurs with guidance from parents as the child learns self-control without feeling shame and doubt. When parents are overly protective or critical, feelings of inferiority will develop.**

24. 1. Although taste influences choices of foods ingested by adolescents, a factor identified in another option generally has more influence over what adolescents eat.
2. Adolescents tend to have few rigid routines because of their busy schedules. A factor identified in another option generally has more influence over what adolescents eat than do routines.
3. **Peers often dictate the dietary choices of adolescents. Fad dieting and demands of socialization that generally involve fast food are common among adolescents.**
4. Although personal preferences may influence choices of foods ingested by adolescents, a factor identified in another option generally has more influence over what adolescents eat.

25. 1. Although sebaceous glands increase in size with age, the amount of sebum produced decreases, hastening the evaporation of water from the stratum corneum and resulting in cracked, dry skin.
2. **Older adults generally experience a deterioration of the hyaline cartilage surface of joints, which tears, allowing bones to be in direct contact with each other. Often this results in the formation of spurs or projecting points that limit joint motion.**
3. Loss of a social support system is a psychosocial, not physiological, change commonly experienced by older adults.
4. **Hearing acuity decreases, particularly in relation to high-pitched sounds, because of atrophy in the organ of Corti and cochlear neurons, loss of sensory hair cells, and degeneration of the stria vascularis.**
5. Older adults have the same need for sleep as younger individuals. However, it is more difficult for older adults to obtain the quality and quantity of sleep desired. Chemical, structural, and functional changes in the nervous system disrupt circadian rhythms and sleep.

26. 1. **The sensorimotor stage (birth to 2 years) is governed by sensations in which simple learning takes place. It progresses from reflex activity, through repetitive behaviors, to imitative behavior. These children are curious, experiment, and learn primarily through trial and error.**
4. **The preoperational stage (2 to 7 years) involves thinking that is concrete and tangible; these children cannot reason beyond the observable. Also, their thinking is transductive; that is, knowledge of one characteristic is transferred to another.**
2. **The concrete-operational stage (7 to 11 years) reflects an increasing ability to use symbols and understand relationships between things and ideas. Judgments are made based on what they reason (conceptual thinking) rather than just what they see (preoperational thinking). Also, they develop the concept of conservation; that is, physical factors (e.g., volume, weight, and number) remain the same even though outward appearances may change.**
3. **The formal operational stage (11 to 15 years) involves thinking that is abstract, theoretical, philosophical, and hypothetical. Thinking is characterized by flexibility, adaptability, and drawing logical conclusions.**

27. 1. Although social isolation is a risk for some older adults because of declining health, death of family members and friends, fear of crime, or injury precipitating a desire not to leave the house, most older adults seek opportunities to maintain and build social contacts via the telephone, Internet, community groups, senior centers, life-care communities, and so on.
2. **Older adults review life experiences and put them all in perspective. With a successful life review, the individual views life as meaningful, respects the self, and feels respect from others.**
3. **The older adult needs to adjust to multiple changes in social roles to emerge emotionally integrated with an intact ego and sense of wholeness.**

Changes in social roles are often dramatic as the result of retirement, death of significant others, changing responsibilities within the extended family structure, moving to different living quarters, and decreasing finances.

4. Although older adults associate with members of all age groups, they generally establish an explicit affiliation with members of their own age group. This supports a sharing of common interests and concerns, as well as meeting belonging and self-esteem needs as older adults seek status among their peers.
5. Older adults do not always have the energy or stamina needed to invest in increasing the number of new meaningful relationships. In addition, they tend to experience a decrease, not increase, in meaningful relationships because of the death of members of their circle of friends and relatives.

28. **1. If sensory overload precipitates anxiety and the autonomic nervous system is stimulated by the fight or flight mechanism, tachycardia will occur.**

2. Sensory overload generally precipitates anxiety, agitation, and restlessness, not drowsiness.
3. **Confusion is a common response to sensory overload. Because of excessive sensory stimulation, a person is unable to perceive the environment accurately or respond appropriately.**
4. **Excessive sensory stimulation from the environment can overwhelm an individual's nervous system resulting in irritability.**
5. Dementia is a progressive irreversible decline in mental function that is not caused by sensory overload.

29. **1. Growth and development comprise an orderly process that follows a predictable, not unpredictable, path. There are three predictable patterns: cephalocaudal—proceeding from head to toe; proximodistal—progressing from gross motor to fine motor movements; and symmetrical—both sides developing equally. Growth is marked by measurable changes in the physical aspects of the life cycle, and development is marked by behavioral changes that occur because of achievement of developmental tasks and their resulting functional abilities and skills.**

2. Growth and development follow a sequential timetable whereby multiple dynamic changes occur in a systematic and orderly manner.
3. Individuals grow and develop in the physiological, cognitive, psychosocial, moral, and spiritual realms in an integrated way, with each one influencing the others.
4. **Growth and development comprise a complex, not simple, process that involves multiple influencing variables, such as genetics, experience, health, culture, and environment.**
5. **The word *static* means stationary, stagnant, or fixed. Growth and development are dynamic and progressive.**

30. **1. A task associated with middle adulthood is sharing of self and performing activities that promote the growth of others, particularly those in the next generation.**

2. Developing peer relationships is one of the developmental tasks of the 6- to 12-year-old child and adolescent, not the middle-aged adult.
3. **A major task of middle adulthood is successfully fulfilling lifelong goals that involve family, career, and society. If these goals are not achieved, a crisis is often precipitated.**
4. Delaying satisfaction is one of the developmental tasks of the 18-month- to 3-year-old child, not the middle-aged adult.
5. Facing death is one of the developmental tasks of the 65-year-old and older adult, not the middle-aged adult.

31. **1. During the school-aged years, children usually grow approximately 2 inches a year and gain 4.5 to 6 lb a year. This child should be assessed further because of the potential for obesity. Obesity in children is increasing in the United States.**

2. Age-appropriate psychosocial development in school-aged children includes associating with peers of the same gender and desiring peer approval. This age group also is developing personal and

interpersonal competence; they are conscientious and industrious.

3. Children approaching 10 to 12 years of age often appear awkward and lanky. They tend to be uncoordinated as muscle and bone growth advances; they are adjusting to these physical changes.
4. Children approaching 10 to 12 years begin to develop a self-image and body image. They have increasing concerns about their appearance and begin to become interested in children of the opposite gender.

32. **1. When a person reaches 60 years of age and older, all physiological systems are less efficient, which reduces compensatory reserve.**

2. In the 40- to 60-year-old age group, a person will begin to see the earliest signs of aging. Changes are gradual and insidious and generally do not have an impact on function.
3. In the 12- to 19-year-old age group, the adolescent is experiencing rapid growth and a beginning transition to adulthood, not a decline in the ability to adapt.
4. In the 3- to 11-year-old age group, children are growing at a continuous pace in their ability to adapt to the world around them, not declining in their ability to adapt.
5. **Infants have immature immune systems and body systems that are still developing. Also, their body's physiological processes have a limited experiential background on which to draw responses to new stressors. These issues result in an inefficiency of adaptation.**

33. 1. This relates to Freud's Anal Stage of development (1 to 3 years). According to Freud, if a parent is strict, overbearing, and oppressive during toilet training, the child may develop traits of an anal retentive personality (e.g., obsessive-compulsive tendencies, rigid thought patterns, stinginess, and/or stubbornness).

2. Seeking excessive attention from others is most likely the result of an unresolved task of the 6- to 12-year-old age group (school age), Industry versus Inferiority. Seeking attention often is an attempt to increase self-esteem.
3. People who have difficulty accepting help from others or who would rather do things themselves generally have not completely resolved the developmental task of infancy, Trust versus Mistrust.
4. **A main developmental task of adolescence is being capable of determining "who you are." An inability to verbalize a sense of self later in life reflects an unresolved conflict of Identity versus Role Confusion.**
5. **A main developmental task of adolescence is forming a sense of personal identity as a foundation for the tasks of young adulthood, making decisions regarding career choices, and selecting a mate. An adult who has difficulty setting goals in life indicates an unresolved conflict of Identity versus Role Confusion.**

34. **1. This statement is a clear example of agism whereby older adults are systematically stereotyped and discriminated against because they are old. This is a form of prejudice, an unfavorable opinion without concrete information about the individual. Agism is based on the misconceptions that older adults are no longer productive, are narrow minded, are unable to learn, are dependent, experience memory loss, live in a nursing home, are ill, are boring, and so on.**

2. **The word *elderly* has a negative connotation. It implies that the person is different from other human beings and is frail, weak, or disabled. To call an adult *cute* is demeaning because it may imply that the person is childlike.**
3. This is not a discriminatory statement indicative of agism.
4. This is not a discriminatory statement indicative of agism.
5. This is not a discriminatory statement indicative of agism.

35. **1. Preschool-aged children have the fine motor skills to open and close zippers and buttons.**

2. **Preschool-aged children have the motor skills necessary to manipulate a toy tool such as a hammer.**

3. **Preschool-aged children have the gross motor skills and balance to be able to hop and skip on one foot, balance on one foot, and perform a broad jump.**
4. Preschool-aged children do not have the strength and balance to ride a two-wheel bicycle. A preschooler usually can ride a tricycle. School-aged children, not preschool-aged children, usually are able to ride a two-wheel bicycle.
5. Preschool-aged children do not have the strength and coordination to swim using the freestyle stroke. Some preschool-aged children are able to do the "doggie paddle." School-aged children, not preschool-aged children, usually are able to swim using the freestyle stroke.

Communication

KEYWORDS

The following words include nursing/medical terminology, concepts, principles, or information relevant to content specifically addressed in the chapter or associated with topics presented in it. English dictionaries, nursing textbooks, and medical dictionaries, such as *Taber's Cyclopedic Medical Dictionary,* are resources that can be used to expand your knowledge and understanding of these words and related information.

Assertive skills
Barriers to communication:
  Advising
  Direct questions
  Disapproving
  False reassurance
  Moralizing
  Patronizing
  Probing
Body language
Communication process:
  Encoding by sender
  Message
  Channels of communication:
    Auditory
    Kinesthetic
    Visual
  Decoding by receiver
  Feedback
Confidential, confidentiality
Confrontation
Congruence
Content themes
Conversation
Empathy, empathetic, empathic
Exploring
Group dynamics
Interaction
Interpersonal communication
Interview:
  Formal
  Informal
Intrapersonal communication
Nonverbal
Rapport
Space:
  Intimate
  Personal
  Social
  Public
Territoriality
Therapeutic communication skills:
  Active listening
  Clarifying
  Focusing
  Indirect question
  Open-ended question
  Paraphrasing
  Reflection
  Responding
  Silence
  Summarizing
  Touching
  Validating
Therapeutic relationship, phases:
  Orientation
  Working
  Termination
Verbal, verbalization

COMMUNICATION: QUESTIONS

1. A nurse is collecting data for an admission nursing history. Which question by the nurse is **best** to open the discussion?
1. "What brought you to the hospital?"
2. "Would it help to discuss your feelings?"
3. "Do you want to talk about your concerns?"
4. "Would you like to talk about why you are here?"

2. A nurse must conduct a focused interview to complete an admission history. Which interviewing technique should the nurse use?
   1. Probing
   2. Clarification
   3. Direct questions
   4. Paraphrasing statements

3. Which statement about communication should the nurse consider to be accurate?
   1. Verbal communication is essential for human relationships.
   2. Hands are the most expressive part of the body.
   3. Behavior clearly reflects feelings.
   4. Communication is inevitable.

4. A patient is extremely upset and mentions something about a work-related issue that the nurse cannot understand. Which is the nurse's **best** response?
   1. "It's natural to worry about your job."
   2. "Your job must be very important to you."
   3. "Calm down so that I can understand what you are saying."
   4. "I'm not quite sure I heard what you were saying about your work."

5. Which is the purpose of the use of humor by a nurse when interacting with a patient?
   1. Diminish feelings of anger
   2. Refocus the patient's attention
   3. Maintain a balanced perspective
   4. Delay dealing with the inevitable

6. A nurse is caring for a patient who is blind in the left eye and visually impaired in the right eye. Which actions should the nurse employ to promote communication with this patient?
   1. Touch the patient's left arm before initiating a conversation
   2. Ensure that the door to the patient's room is on the patient's left side
   3. Close the window curtains and dim the lights before speaking with the patient
   4. Knock on the door and request permission to enter before approaching the patient

7. A patient is admitted to the hospital with cirrhosis of the liver caused by long-term alcohol abuse. Which is the **best** response by the nurse when the patient says, "I really don't believe that my drinking a couple of beers a day has anything to do with my liver problem"?
   1. "You find it hard to believe that beer can hurt the liver."
   2. "How long is it that you have been drinking several beers a day?"
   3. "Each beer is equivalent to one shot of liquor so it's just as damaging to the liver as hard liquor."
   4. "Do you believe that beer is not harmful even though research shows that it is just as bad for you as hard liquor?"

8. Which is being communicated when the nurse leans forward during a patient interview?
   1. Aggression
   2. Anxiety
   3. Interest
   4. Privacy

9. Which statement describes the following proverb? *What you do speaks so loudly I cannot hear what you say.*
   1. Hearing ability is an important factor in communicating.
   2. Nonverbal messages are often more meaningful than words.
   3. Listening to what people say requires attention to what is being said.
   4. When people talk too loudly it is hard to understand what is being said.

10. A mother whose young daughter has died of leukemia is crying and is unable to talk about her feelings. Which is the **best** response by the nurse?
    1. "Everyone will remember her because she was so cute. She was one of our favorites."
    2. "As hard as this is, it is probably for the best because she was in a lot of pain."
    3. "She put up the good fight but now she is out of pain and in heaven."
    4. "It must be hard to deal with such a precious loss."

11. A young adult who had a leg amputated because of trauma says, "No one will ever choose to love a person with one leg." Which is the **best** response by the nurse?
    1. "You are a good-looking person, and you will have no trouble meeting someone who cares."
    2. "You may feel that way now, but you will feel differently as time passes."
    3. "Do you feel that no one will marry you because you have one leg?"
    4. "How do you see your situation at this point?"

12. A nurse is changing a patient's dressing over an abdominal wound. Which level of space around the patient is entered during the dressing change?
    1. Public
    2. Social
    3. Intimate
    4. Personal

13. Which stage of an interview establishes the relationship between the nurse and the patient?
    1. Preinteraction stage
    2. Orientation stage
    3. Examining stage
    4. Working stage

14. A patient is exhibiting anxious behavior and states, "I just found out that I have cancer everywhere and I don't have very long to live. My life is over." Which is the **best** response by the nurse?
    1. "It might be good if your family were here right now. Shall I call them?"
    2. "What might be the best way to approach this terrible news?"
    3. "That is so sad. You must feel like crying."
    4. "It sounds like you feel hopeless."

15. Which interviewing skill is used when the nurse says, "You mentioned before that you are having a problem with your colostomy."
    1. Focusing
    2. Clarifying
    3. Paraphrasing
    4. Acknowledging

16. A patient says, "I am really nervous about having a spinal tap tomorrow." Which is the **best** response by the nurse?
    1. "I'll ask the doctor for a little medication to help you relax."
    2. "Patients who have had a spinal tap say it is not that uncomfortable."
    3. "It's all right to be nervous, and I don't remember anyone who wasn't."
    4. "Your physician is excellent and is very careful when spinal taps are done."

17. A patient with chest pain is being admitted to the emergency department. When asked about next of kin the patient states, "Don't bother calling my daughter; she is always too busy." Which is the **best** response by the nurse?
    1. "She might be upset if you don't call her."
    2. "What does your daughter do that makes her so busy?"
    3. "Is there someone else that you would like me to call for you?"
    4. "I can't imagine that your daughter wouldn't want to know that you are sick."

18. Which is the nurse doing when using the interviewing technique of *attentive listening*?
    1. Identifying the patient's concerns and exploring them with why questions
    2. Determining the content and feeling of the patient's message
    3. Employing silence to encourage the patient to talk
    4. Using nonverbal skills to display interest

19. A patient who has had a number of postoperative complications appears upset and agitated, yet withdrawn. Which is the **most** appropriate statement by the nurse?
    1. "You seem distressed. Tell me why you are upset."
    2. "You've been having a pretty rough time of it since surgery."
    3. "It's not uncommon to have complications after the kind of surgery that you had."
    4. "I'm not sure that I know everything that has been happening. Tell me what has happened to you since surgery."

20. A nurse is admitting a patient to the unit who was transferred from the emergency department. Which should the nurse do to facilitate communication?
    1. Ensure that the patient has an effective way to communicate with health-care team members.
    2. Use interviewing techniques to control the direction of the patient's communication.
    3. Minimize energy spent by the patient on negative feelings and concerns.
    4. Refocus to the positive aspects of the patient's situation and prognosis.

21. A nurse is caring for a confused patient with a diagnosis of dementia of the Alzheimer's type. Which should the nurse say when assisting the patient to eat?
    1. "Please eat your meat."
    2. "It's important that you eat."
    3. "What would you like to eat?"
    4. "If you don't eat, you can't have dessert."

22. A patient states, "Do you think I could have cancer?" The nurse responds, "What did the doctor tell you?" Which interviewing approach did the nurse use?
    1. Paraphrasing
    2. Confrontation
    3. Reflective technique
    4. Open-ended question

23. A nurse is developing a therapeutic relationship with a patient with emotional needs. Which nursing interventions are essential during the working stage of the relationship?
    1. Establish a formal or informal contract that addresses the patient's problems.
    2. Implement nursing actions that are designed to achieve expected patient outcomes.
    3. Develop rapport and trust so the patient feels protected and an initial plan can be identified.
    4. Clearly identify the role of the nurse and establish the parameters of the professional relationship.

24. A nurse uses reflective technique when communicating with an anxious patient. On which does the nurse focus when using reflective technique in this situation?
    1. Feelings
    2. Content themes
    3. Clarification of information
    4. Summarization of the topics discussed

25. A patient states, "My wife is going to be very upset that my prostate surgery probably is going to leave me impotent." Which is the **best** response by the nurse?
   1. "I'm sure your wife will be willing to make this sacrifice in exchange for your well-being."
   2. "The surgeons are getting great results with nerve-sparing surgery today."
   3. "Your wife may not put as much emphasis on sex as you think."
   4. "Let's talk about how you feel about this surgery."

26. A patient states, "I think that I am dying." The nurse responds, "You believe that you are dying?" Which interviewing approach did the nurse use?
   1. Focusing
   2. Reflecting
   3. Validating
   4. Paraphrasing

27. A nurse plans to foster a therapeutic relationship with a patient. Which is important for the nurse to do?
   1. Work on establishing a friendship with the patient.
   2. Use humor to defuse emotionally charged topics of discussion.
   3. Sympathize with the patient when the patient shares sad feelings.
   4. Demonstrate respect when discussing emotionally charged subjects.

28. A patient appears tearful and is quiet and withdrawn. The nurse says, "You seem very sad today." Which interviewing approach did the nurse use?
   1. Examining
   2. Reflecting
   3. Clarifying
   4. Orienting

29. A patient is admitted to the hospital with a tentative medical diagnosis and multiple diagnostic tests are performed. Where in the patient's chart can the nurse find documentation about the current medical diagnosis after the diagnostic test results are reviewed by the primary health-care provider?
   1. Progress Notes
   2. Admission Sheet
   3. History and Physical
   4. Social Service Record

30. Which nursing actions should the nurse implement when speaking with an older adult whose hearing is impaired? **Select all that apply.**
   1. _____Limit background noise.
   2. _____Exaggerate lip movements.
   3. _____Lower the pitch of your voice.
   4. _____Stand directly in front of the patient when speaking.
   5. _____Raise the volume of your voice while speaking directly toward the patient's good ear.

31. A patient with a colostomy wants to learn how to irrigate a newly created colostomy. The nurse provides this teaching by developing a therapeutic nurse-patient relationship and implementing teaching strategies. Identify the statements that are included in the working stage of this therapeutic relationship. **Select all that apply.**
   1. _____"How do you feel about doing this procedure?"
   2. _____"Would you like to try to insert the cone yourself today?"
   3. _____"You did a great job managing the instillation of fluid today."
   4. _____"I am here to help you learn how to irrigate your colostomy."
   5. _____"I'll arrange for a home care nurse to visit you in your home when you are discharged."

32. A risk manager is conducting a retrospective audit of a patient's clinical record to identify the use of unacceptable abbreviations. Which abbreviations did the risk manager identify that are on The Joint Commission's official *Do Not Use List*? **Select all that apply.**

1. _____U
2. _____cc
3. _____mg
4. _____MS
5. _____QOD
6. _____0800 hour

Medication Administration Record
MS 4 mg subcutaneous at 1400 hour and patient verbalized relief within 15 minutes. Patient serum glucose was 180 at 1700 hour; 4 U regular insulin administered subcutaneously as prescribed.

Intake and Output Record
0800 Hour: Milk 60 cc, orange juice 120 cc; coffee 120 cc

Progress Note
Patient to be discharged in a.m. and will receive physical therapy QOD.

33. A nurse is attempting to develop a helping relationship with a patient who was recently diagnosed with cancer. Which factors are unique to this helping relationship? **Select all that apply.**

1. _____The patient is permitted to assume the dominant role.
2. _____The nurse and the patient equally share information.
3. _____The interaction is specific to the patient.
4. _____The interaction is guided by a purpose.
5. _____The needs of both participants are met.

34. A nurse is using military time when entering information into a patient's clinical record. For example, the clock below indicates that the time is 0708 a.m. Which number in military time should the nurse enter to document a wound irrigation that was implemented at 9 p.m.?

1. 0900
2. 1900
3. 2100
4. 2300

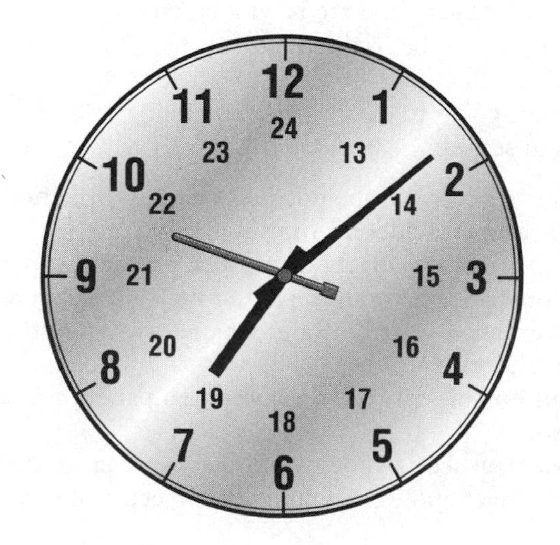

35. An agitated 80-year-old patient states, "I'm having trouble with my bowels." Which responses by the nurse incorporate the interviewing skill of paraphrasing? **Select all that apply.**
1. _____"You're having trouble with your bowels?"
2. _____"It sounds like your bowels are causing you problems."
3. _____"You sound upset that your bowels are causing difficulties."
4. _____"It's common to have problems with the bowels at your age."
5. _____"When did you first notice having trouble with your bowels?"

36. A patient states, "I can't believe that I couldn't even eat half my breakfast." Which statements by the nurse use the interviewing skill of reflection? **Select all that apply.**
1. _____"Let's talk about your inability to eat."
2. _____"What part of your breakfast were you able to eat?"
3. _____"You appear startled that you did not finish your tray of food."
4. _____"How long have you been unable to eat most of your breakfast?"
5. _____"You seem surprised that you were unable to eat all your breakfast."

37. A nurse in a sub-acute unit in a skilled nursing facility is caring for a patient who recently had the surgical creation of a colostomy. Place the following nursing actions in the order that reflects the nurse-patient communication process, beginning with the first stage and progressing to the last stage.
1. Provide positive feedback to the patient for successful performance of a colostomy irrigation.
2. Assist the patient to learn how to perform colostomy self-care.
3. Review all the information on the patient's clinical record.
4. Explore the reasons for the nurse-patient interaction.
5. Summarize the goals and objectives achieved.
6. Introduce self to the patient.

Answer: _______________

38. Which abilities of the nurse are important to achieve effective therapeutic communication? **Select all that apply.**
1. _____Using interviewing skills
2. _____Remaining nonjudgmental
3. _____Sending just verbal messages
4. _____Being assertive when collecting data
5. _____Displaying sympathy when communicating

39. A patient is to have arthroscopic surgery of the knee to repair a torn tendon. The patient says, "I don't know if I'll make it through this surgery." Which responses by the nurse may block further communication by the patient? **Select all that apply.**
1. _____"The type of surgery you are having is minor."
2. _____"Surgery often can be frightening."
3. _____"Everything will be all right."
4. _____"You are not going to die."
5. _____"You sound scared."

40. Which should a nurse never do when documenting information on a patient's electronic medical record? **Select all that apply.**
1. _____Leave the patient's medical record open on the computer screen when entering the patient's room to administer a medication.
2. _____Share information verbally about a patient with another nurse who is also caring for the patient.
3. _____Document nursing care administered to a patient immediately after it is completed.
4. _____Give a personal access code to another member of the health-care team.
5. _____Document exact quotes of a patient's subjective information.

COMMUNICATION: ANSWERS AND RATIONALES

1. **1. This is a focused open-ended statement that invites the patient to communicate while centering on the reason for seeking health care.**
2. This direct question can be answered with a "yes" or "no" response. If the response is "no," then communication will be cut off.
3. This direct question can be answered with a "yes" or "no" response, which may limit communication.
4. This direct question can be answered with a "yes" or "no" response. The patient may not like to talk but the patient may need to talk.

2. 1. Probing questions violate the patient's privacy, may cut off communication, and are inappropriate even in a focused interview. Probing interviewing occurs when the nurse persistently attempts to obtain information even after the patient indicates an unwillingness to discuss the topic or the nurse pursues information out of curiosity, rather than because the information is significant.
2. Although clarification may be used during a focused interview to understand what the patient is saying, it is not the primary technique used for seeking specific information.
3. A focused interview explores a particular topic or obtains specific information. Direct questions meet these objectives and avoid extraneous information.
4. Paraphrasing may be used during a focused interview to redirect ideas back to the patient so that the patient can verify that the nurse received the message accurately or to allow the patient to hear what was said. However, it is not a technique that obtains specific information quickly.

3. 1. All communication, not just verbal communication, is essential for human relationships.
2. The face, not the hands, is the most expressive part of the body.
3. Behavior may imply, not clearly reflect, feelings. The nurse should obtain verbal feedback from the patient regarding assumptions about behavior.
4. Theory indicates that all behavior has meaning, people are always behaving, and we cannot stop behaving or communicating; therefore, communication is inevitable.

4. 1. This may or may not be an accurate assumption.
2. This makes an assumption that may be erroneous.
3. This patronizing response treats the patient in a condescending manner. The patient cannot calm down.
4. This response requests additional information in an attempt to clarify an unclear message.

5. 1. Humor used inappropriately can cause anger to be increased, suppressed, or repressed. Anger should be expressed safely, not diminished.
2. The focus should be on the patient's concerns.
3. Humor is an interpersonal tool and a healing strategy. It releases physical and psychic energy, enhances well-being, reduces anxiety, increases pain tolerance, and places experiences within the context of life.
4. Coping strategies should not be delayed because delay increases stress and anxiety and prolongs the process.

6. 1. Touching a patient with a visual impairment before speaking is an intrusive action and may startle the patient.
2. A door to the room on the patient's left side will require the patient to completely turn the head to the left so that the patient can use the right eye to view a person entering the room. The door should be on the patient's right side.
3. Patients with visual impairments may still have some sight. Adequate lighting facilitates nonverbal communication.
4. Knocking on the door before entering the room alerts the patient to the fact that someone is at the door and requesting permission to enter the room demonstrates respect and provides for privacy.

7. **1. This is an example of paraphrasing. It repeats the content in the patient's message in similar words to provide feedback to let the patient know whether the message was understood and to prompt further communication.**

2. This response does not address the content or emotional theme of the patient's statement. In addition, this probing question may be a barrier to further communication.
3. Although factual, this response is confrontational. This nurse's statement may put the patient on the defensive and inhibit further communication.
4. This assertive, confronting, judgmental response may put the patient on the defensive and cut off communication.

8. 1. Piercing eye contact, increased voice volume, challenging or confrontational conversation, invasion of personal space, and inappropriate touching convey aggression, which is a hostile, injurious, or destructive action or manner.
2. A closed posture, avoidance of eye contact, increased muscle tension, and increased motor activity convey anxiety.
3. Leaning forward is a nonverbal behavior that conveys involvement. It is a form of physical attending, which is being present to another.
4. Privacy is not reflected by leaning forward during an interview. Privacy is facilitated by pulling a patient's curtain or finding a separate room or quiet space to talk.

9. 1. Although hearing, one aspect of decoding a message, is an important factor in the communication process, it is unrelated to the stated proverb.
2. Nonverbal communication (e.g., body language) conveys messages without words and is under less conscious control than verbal statements. When a person's words and behavior are incongruent, nonverbal behavior most likely reflects the person's true feelings.
3. Although this true statement reflects active listening, it is unrelated to the stated proverb.
4. This statement is unrelated to the stated proverb. The volume of a message may or may not influence understanding of the message. The volume of a message occurs on the physiological level, whereas understanding a message occurs on the cognitive level.

10. 1. This response is not therapeutic because it focuses on the nurse rather than on the mother.
2. The first part of this response minimizes the loss. The second part of the response focuses on the pain experienced by the child, which may increase the mother's grief.
3. This response minimizes the loss and focuses on the pain experienced by the child, which may increase the mother's grief. Also, the mother may not believe in heaven.
4. The nurse's response is empathetic. The response focuses on the feelings surrounding the loss and provides an opportunity for the mother to verbalize.

11. 1. This negates the patient's concerns and provides false reassurance. The patient needs to focus on the "negative" before focusing on the "positive." In addition, only the future will tell if the patient meets someone who cares.
2. This is false reassurance. There is no way the nurse can ensure that this belief will change.
3. This is an example of paraphrasing, which restates the patient's message in similar words. It promotes communication.
4. This statement is unnecessary. The patient has already stated a point of view.

12. 1. Touching is not used with public distance. Public space (12 feet and beyond) is effective for communicating with groups or the community. Individuality is lost.
2. Invasive touching does not occur with social distance. Social space (4 to 12 feet) is effective for more formal interactions or group conversations.
3. Physically caring for a patient involves inspection and touch that invades the instinctual, protective distance immediately surrounding an individual. Intimate space (physical contact to 1½ feet) is characterized by body contact and visual exposure.
4. "Laying on of the hands" does not occur with personal distance. Personal space (1½ to 4 feet) is effective for communicating with another. It is close enough to imply caring and is not extended to the distance that implies lack of involvement.

13. 1. The preinteraction stage occurs before the nurse meets the patient. During this stage the nurse gathers information about the patient.
2. The purposes of the orientation stage of an interview are to establish rapport and orient the interviewee. A relationship is

established through a process of creating goodwill and trust. The orientation stage focuses on explaining the purpose and nature of the interview and what is expected of the patient.

3. There is no stage called the examining stage in an interview. Examining takes place during a physical assessment, when specific skills are used to collect data systematically to identify health problems.
4. This is not the purpose of the working stage. In the working stage, also called the body stage, of an interview patients communicate how they think, feel, know, and perceive in response to questions by the nurse.

14. 1. This response abdicates the nurse's responsibility to explore the patient's concerns immediately. In addition, it could be an erroneous assumption.
2. The patient is in the shock and disbelief mode of coping and will not be able to explore approaches to coping. In addition, using the words "terrible news" may increase anxiety and hopelessness.
3. This response imposes the nurse's feelings and own coping skills into the situation.
4. This is an example of reflective technique because the nurse incorporated the patient's feelings into the response. When no solutions to a problem are evident, a person becomes hopeless (i.e., despairing, despondent).

15. 1. This example of focusing helps the patient explore a topic of importance. The nurse selects one topic for further discussion from among several topics presented by the patient.
2. This is not an example of clarifying, which lets the patient know that a message was unclear and seeks specific information to make the message clearer.
3. This is not an example of paraphrasing, which is restating the patient's message in similar words.
4. This is not an example of acknowledging, which is providing nonjudgmental recognition for a contribution to the conversation, a change in behavior, or an effort by the patient.

16. 1. This statement avoids the patient's feelings and fails to respond to the patient's need to talk about concerns. It cuts off communication.
2. This is a generalization that minimizes the patient's concern and should be avoided.
3. This statement is therapeutic. It recognizes the patient's feelings, gives the patient permission to feel nervous, and reassures the patient that one's behavior is not unusual. This statement sets the groundwork for the next statement, such as, "Let's talk a little bit about the spinal tap and the concerns you may have."
4. This is false reassurance, which discourages discussion of feelings and should be avoided.

17. 1. This response will put the patient on the defensive and jeopardize the nurse-patient relationship.
2. This response requires the patient to rationalize the daughter's behavior and focuses on information that is not significant at this time.
3. This response lets the patient know that the message has been heard and moves forward to meet the need to notify a significant other of the patient's situation.
4. This provides false reassurance. Only the daughter can convey this message.

18. 1. "Why" statements are direct questions that tend to put the patient on the defensive and cut off communication.
2. Attentive listening is the active use of all the senses to comprehend and appreciate the patient's verbal and nonverbal thoughts and feelings.
3. Silence is a passive interaction. Silence allows the patient time for quiet contemplation of what has been discussed.
4. When talking with patients, verbal and nonverbal cues are used to indicate care and concern, which promote communication.

19. 1. The first part of this statement uses the therapeutic interviewing technique of reflection, which identifies the underlying feelings of the patient and is appropriate. However, the second half of the statement is asking for an explanation, which is inappropriate. Patients often interpret "why" questions as accusations, which can cause resentment and mistrust and should be avoided.
2. This is an example of the therapeutic interviewing skill of an open-ended statement. It demonstrates that the nurse recognizes what the patient is

going through, and the statement encourages free verbalization by the patient. At the very least it demonstrates caring and concern.
3. This statement minimizes the patient's feelings and is not supportive.
4. This statement will not inspire confidence in the nurse. Nurses should know what is happening if care is to be comprehensive and patient centered.

20. **1. Communication between the patient and health-care providers is essential, particularly for obtaining subjective data and feedback. Speech, pantomime, writing, touch, and picture boards are examples of channels of transmission (i.e., media used to convey a message).**
2. The patient, not the nurse, should direct the flow of communication.
3. Negative feelings or concerns must be addressed. Both physical and psychic energy are used when coping with stress.
4. The focus must be on the patient's present concerns before refocusing to other issues because anxiety increases if immediate concerns are not addressed. Focusing on the negative sometimes is necessary before focusing on the positive.

21. **1. Confused patients more easily understand simple words and sentences.**
2. This may not be understood by the confused patient because the word "important" involves a conceptual thought. These patients respond better to concrete communication.
3. A confused patient may not be able to make a decision.
4. This is a threat and should be avoided when talking with patients. Also, it involves interpreting a "cause and effect" relationship.

22. 1. The nurse's response is not an example of paraphrasing, which is restating the patient's basic message in similar words.
2. This is not an example of confrontation. A confronting or challenging statement fails to consider feelings, puts the patient on the defensive, and is a barrier to communication.
3. The nurse's response is not an example of reflective technique, which is referring back the basic feelings underlying the patient's statement.
4. This open-ended statement invites the patient to elaborate on the expressed thought with more than a one- or two-word response.

23. 1. Formal or informal contracts are established during the introductory (orientation), not working, stage of a therapeutic relationship.
2. During the working stage of the therapeutic relationship, nursing interventions have a twofold purpose: assisting patients to explore and understand their thoughts and feelings and facilitating and supporting patients' decisions and actions.
3. The development of trust is the primary goal of the introductory (orientation), not working, stage of a therapeutic relationship. Trust is achieved through respect, concern, credibility, and reliability.
4. These tasks are achieved during the introductory (orientation), not working, stage of a therapeutic relationship.

24. **1. Reflective technique requires active listening to identify the underlying emotional concerns or feelings contained in patients' messages. These feelings are then referred back to patients to promote a clearer understanding of what they have said.**
2. Content themes are referred back to patients through paraphrasing, which is a restatement of what was said in similar words.
3. When seeking clarification, the nurse can indicate confusion, restate the message, or ask the patient to elaborate in an attempt to make the patient's message more clearly understood.
4. Summarization is not reflective technique. Summarization reviews the significant points of the discussion to reiterate or clarify information.

25. 1. This response is false reassurance. Only the wife can make this statement.
2. Although a true statement, this response negates the patient's concerns and cuts off communication.
3. This may or may not be a true statement. Only the wife can make this statement.
4. The patient may be using projection to cope with the potential for impotence. This response indicates that it is acceptable to talk about sexuality and invites the patient to verbalize concerns.

26. 1. This is not an example of focusing, which centers on the key elements of the patient's message in an attempt to eliminate vagueness. It keeps a rambling conversation on target to explore the major concern. The patient was not rambling.
2. This is not an example of reflecting, which focuses on feelings.
3. This is not an example of validating. Consensual validation, a form of clarification, verifies the meaning of specific words rather than the overall meaning of the message. This ensures that both patient and nurse agree on the meaning of the words used.
4. The nurse's response is an example of paraphrasing because it uses similar words to restate the patient's message.

27. 1. The nurse should maintain a professional relationship with the patient. Nurses may be "friendly" toward patients but should not establish a "friendship" with a patient.
2. Humor with emotionally charged issues may be viewed as minimizing concerns or being frivolous and could be a barrier to communication.
3. Sympathy denotes pity, which should be avoided. The nurse should empathize, not sympathize, with the patient.
4. Emotionally charged topics should be approached with respectful, sincere interactions that are accepting and nonjudgmental and that will promote further verbalizations.

28. 1. Examining is not an interviewing technique.
2. Reflective technique refers to feelings implied in the content of verbal communication or in exhibited nonverbal behaviors. Patients who are crying, quiet, and withdrawn often are sad.
3. This is not an example of clarifying, which is the use of a statement to understand a message better when communication is unclear, rambling, or garbled.
4. This is not an example of orienting. Reality orientation is a nursing technique used to assist patients in restoring an awareness of what is actual, authentic, or real.

29. 1. Generally, the Progress Notes contain documentation by all members of the health-care team. After a patient is admitted and diagnostic tests are completed, the patient's medical diagnosis may change. The ongoing changes and current status of the patient are documented in the Progress Notes.
2. The Admission Sheet is the best source for identifying the patient's admitting medical diagnosis, but it will not contain the current medical diagnosis if the diagnosis changed after completion of diagnostic tests.
3. The History and Physical Examination contain a history of the patient, results of the physical examination, and a list of the medical problems on the day of admission to the hospital. The admission medical diagnosis may be different after diagnostic tests are completed.
4. Although the patient's medical diagnosis might be documented on the patient's Social Service Record, it is not the major source for this information.

30. 1. Limiting competing stimuli promotes reception of verbal messages.
2. Exaggerating lip movements may be demeaning and ineffective because the patient may not be able to read lips.
3. Lowering the pitch of the voice may be helpful. Hearing loss in the older adult typically involves a decreased perception of high-pitched sounds.
4. Standing directly in front of the patient when speaking focuses the patient's attention on the nurse. A hearing-impaired receiver must be aware that a message is being sent before the message can be received and decoded.
5. Raising the volume of the voice is demeaning and may be viewed by the patient as aggressive behavior.

31. 1. This statement reflects the orientation stages of a therapeutic relationship. Although exploration of feelings is done throughout the stages, the primary goal of the orientation stage is the establishment of trust. Trust is promoted when the nurse focuses on the patient's emotional needs, is respectful, and individualizes care.
2. This statement reflects the working stage of a therapeutic relationship. It involves completing interventions that address expected outcomes, such as learning how to perform a colostomy irrigation.
3. This statement reflects the working stage of a therapeutic relationship. It

includes providing feedback and encouragement.

4. This statement reflects the orientation stage of a therapeutic relationship. The nurse and patient make a verbal agreement to work together to assist the patient to achieve a goal.
5. This statement reflects the termination stage of a therapeutic relationship. It focuses on summarizing what has transpired and been accomplished and looks to the future.

32. 1. The abbreviations U and u for *units* are on The Joint Commission's official *Do Not Use List*. These abbreviations may be mistaken for the number 0, the number 4, or cc. The word *unit* should be written out in full.

2. An abbreviation for *cubic centimeters* is cc. The abbreviation cc is not on The Joint Commission's official *Do Not Use List*. However, it is being considered for future inclusion because it can be confused with the word *units* when written poorly. The use of milliliters in place of cc is preferred by The Joint Commission.
3. The use of the abbreviation mg for *milligram* is not on The Joint Commission's official *Do Not Use List*.
4. **The abbreviation MS for *morphine sulfate* is on The Joint Commission's official *Do Not Use List*. MS can be mistaken for *morphine sulfate* or *magnesium sulfate*. The name of the medication should be spelled out in full.**
5. **The use of the abbreviation QOD for every other day is on The Joint Commission's official *Do Not Use List*. Other abbreviations for every other day include qod, q.o.d., and QOD, and they are also on The Joint Commission's official *Do Not Use List*. "Every other day" should be written out in full.**
6. The use of 0800 represents 8 a.m. in military time. This reflects acceptable documentation.

33. 1. There are times that the nurse, not the patient, must assume a dominant role; examples include when the patient is unconscious, out of touch with reality, in a crisis, or experiencing panic.

2. In a therapeutic relationship, the focus is on the patient, not the nurse.
3. **The helping relationship (interpersonal relationship, therapeutic relationship) is a personal, patient-focused, process. The patient is the center of the health team and therefore the focus of any nurse-patient interaction.**
4. **Nursing interventions should be designed to achieve desirable patient outcomes. Nursing care is purposeful and goal directed.**
5. The purpose of a therapeutic relationship is to focus on and meet the needs of the patient, not the nurse.

34. 1. 0900 is 9 a.m.

2. 1900 is 7 p.m.
3. **2100 is 9 p.m. The large font numbers reflect a.m. The small font numbers reflect p.m.**
4. 2300 is 11 p.m.

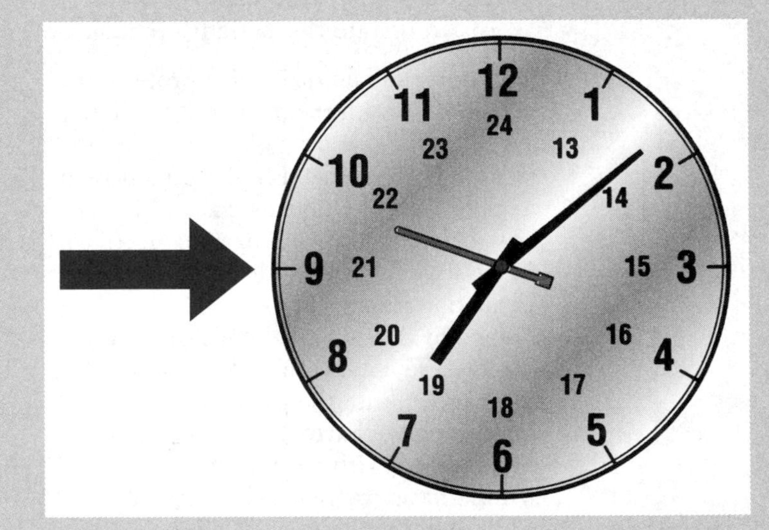

35. 1. A nurse uses the technique of paraphrasing when restating a patient's comment or using similar words to rephrase what the patient has said.

2. **The nurse's statement substitutes the word *problems* for *trouble*, which paraphrases the patient's comment.**
3. This is not an example of paraphrasing. This statement uses the interviewing technique of reflection because it focuses on feelings rather than words.
4. This negates the patient's concern and shuts off communication.
5. This is not an example of paraphrasing; it is a direct question that collects specific information.

36. 1. The nurse's response does not employ reflective technique. This open-ended statement invites the patient to explore factors that may be influencing eating.

2. This response is an example of a direct question, not the use of reflective technique. It elicits a minimal amount of

information about only one aspect of eating.

3. **This statement is an example of reflective technique because it focuses on the feeling of being startled.**
4. This response is an example of a direct question, not the use of reflective technique.
5. **This statement is an example of reflective technique because it focuses on the feeling of surprise.**

37. **3. During the *preinteraction stage* of the communication process, the nurse gathers information about the patient. This stage occurs before meeting the patient.**

6. During the *orientation stage* of the communication process, the nurse introduces himself or herself to the patient and begins to establish a rapport with the patient.

4. During the *orientation stage* of the communication process, the nurse and patient exchange information, clarify roles, and identify goals and objectives of the interaction.

2. During the *working stage* of the communication process, the nurse and patient work toward meeting the patient's needs. The nurse may function as a caregiver, counselor, teacher, resource person, etc.

1. During the *working stage* of the communication process, the nurse provides feedback about the patient's performance.

5. During the *termination stage* of the communication process, the nurse summarizes what has been accomplished, reinforces past learning, arranges for available resources, and concludes the interpersonal relationship.

38.
1. **Communication is facilitated by interviewing techniques that involve attitudes, behaviors, and verbal messages. Interviewing skills promote therapeutic communication because they are patient centered and goal directed.**
2. **A nonjudgmental attitude communicates acceptance to the patient, which provides emotional support and precipitates further communication.**
3. Communication involves both verbal and nonverbal messages. Often nonverbal messages carry more meaning than verbal messages because actions speak louder than words.
4. Assertiveness when collecting data may be perceived by the patient as aggression, which is a barrier to communication.
5. A therapeutic relationship should avoid sympathy because it implies pity. The nurse should empathize, not sympathize, with patients.

39.
1. **This response minimizes the patient's concerns. It is not minor surgery for this patient.**
2. This example of reflective technique focuses on feelings, which promotes communication.
3. **This response is false reassurance. It denies the patient's concerns about survival and does not invite the patient to elaborate.**
4. **This response denies the patient's feelings and is false reassurance. Also, it closes communication and does not provide the patient with an opportunity to discuss concerns.**
5. This example of reflective technique identifies feelings, which promotes communication.

40.
1. **Leaving the patient's medical record open on the computer screen violates patient confidentiality as well as leaves the file vulnerable to another person contaminating the information in the file.**
2. A nurse should communicate, verbally and in writing, important information to other members of the health-care team responsible for caring for the patient. Valuable time may lapse before other members of the team read the patient's electronic medical record.
3. Documenting care immediately after it is administered ensures that the information is in the patient's medical record. Also, delaying documentation may result in the nurse's forgetting to include pertinent information.
4. **This ensures that only the nurse assigned the code can insert information into the electronic medical record via that code. This protects the nurse who has the code.**
5. Inclusion of exact patient statements prevents the nurse from including personal interpretations that may not be accurate.

Psychological Support

KEYWORDS

The following words include nursing/medical terminology, concepts, principles, and information relevant to content specifically addressed in the chapter or associated with topics presented in it. English dictionaries, nursing textbooks, and medical dictionaries, such as *Taber's Cyclopedic Medical Dictionary,* are resources that can be used to expand your knowledge and understanding of these words and related information.

Anxiety:
- Mild
- Moderate
- Severe
- Panic, panic attack

Behavior modification
Beliefs
Bereavement
Body image
Confusion
Conscious, unconscious, subconscious
Coping
Crisis:
- Adventitious/unpredictable events
- Developmental/maturational
- Situational

Crisis intervention
Defense mechanisms:
- Compensation
- Conversion
- Denial
- Depersonalization
- Dissociation
- Identification
- Intellectualization
- Introjection
- Minimization
- Projection
- Rationalization
- Reaction formation
- Regression
- Repression
- Sublimation
- Substitution
- Suppression

Delirium
Delusions
Dementia
Dependence
Depression
Desensitization
Ego integrity
Egocentric
Empathy, empathetic, empathic
Freudian terms:
- Ego
- Id
- Superego

Grieving:
- Anticipatory
- Dysfunctional
- Stages of grieving (Kübler-Ross):
  - Denial
  - Anger
  - Bargaining
  - Depression
  - Acceptance

Guided imagery
Hallucinations
Hopelessness
Meditation
Memory
Midlife crisis
Personal identity
Positive mental attitude
Powerlessness
Progressive relaxation
Psychodynamic
Psychosocial development
Psychotherapy
Role:
- Role ambiguity
- Role conflict
- Role strain

Self-concept
Self-esteem
Social isolation
Spirituality, spiritual distress
Suicide, suicidal
Sympathy
Transference/countertransference
Trust
Values

PSYCHOLOGICAL SUPPORT: QUESTIONS

1. A patient with a terminal illness tells the nurse, "I have lived a long life. I am ready to go." Which is the nurse's **best** response?
1. Offer the patient a back rub.
2. Sit quietly by the patient's bedside.
3. Tell the family about the patient's statement.
4. Discuss with the patient how dying is part of the life cycle.

2. A man with a heart condition continues to perform strenuous sports against medical advice. Which defense mechanism does the nurse identify the patient is using?
1. Denial
2. Repression
3. Introjection
4. Dissociation

3. Which is an important concept to consider about anxiety to provide appropriate nursing care?
1. Panic attacks generally have a slow onset that can be prevented if identified early.
2. One can conceptualize anxiety as being similar to the health-illness continuum.
3. People who lead healthy lifestyles rarely experience anxiety.
4. Anxiety is an abnormal reaction to realistic danger.

4. Which word reflects the ability of a person to perceive another person's emotions accurately?
1. Trust
2. Empathy
3. Sympathy
4. Autonomy

5. What is the consequence when the nurse denies a patient the use of a defense mechanism?
1. Causes more anxiety
2. Precipitates withdrawal
3. Facilitates effective coping
4. Encourages emotional growth

6. Which defense mechanism is being used when a patient who has just been diagnosed with terminal cancer calmly says to the nurse, "I'll have to get on the Internet to assess my options"?
1. Intellectualization
2. Introjection
3. Depression
4. Denial

7. A patient is told that surgery is necessary and the patient begins to experience elevations in pulse, respirations, and blood pressure. Which stage of anxiety is indicated by these nursing assessments?
1. Mild
2. Moderate
3. Severe
4. Panic

8. A nurse concludes that a woman is remembering only the good times after the death of her husband. Which defense mechanism is the woman using?
1. Compensation
2. Minimization
3. Repression
4. Regression

9. A patient strongly states the desire to go to the hospital coffee shop for lunch regardless of hospital policy. Which does the nurse conclude that this behavior **most** likely reflects?
   1. Anger with the policies of the hospital
   2. Dissatisfaction with hospital meals
   3. The need to regain a little control
   4. A desire for a change of scenery

10. A nurse is teaching a patient about the positive effects of exercise to reduce anxiety. Which patient comment about how exercise reduces anxiety indicates that the patient understands the nurse's teaching?
   1. "It stimulates the production of endorphins."
   2. "It interferes with the ability to concentrate."
   3. "It reduces the metabolism of epinephrine."
   4. "It decreases the acidity of blood."

11. A primary health-care provider informs a patient that the diagnosis is inoperable cancer and the prognosis is poor. After the primary health-care provider leaves the room, the patient begins to cry. Which should the nurse do?
   1. Touch the patient's hand to provide support.
   2. Leave the room to give the patient privacy to cry.
   3. Telephone the patient's family to inform them of the diagnosis.
   4. Ask the patient questions to encourage a ventilation of feelings.

12. A nurse is caring for a patient who is scheduled for intravenous chemotherapy for cancer. Which defense mechanism is being used when the patient says to the daughter, "Be brave"?
   1. Rationalization
   2. Minimization
   3. Substitution
   4. Projection

13. A patient says to a nurse, "I'm the same age as my father when he died. Am I going to die of my cancer?" Which is the appropriate inference about what the patient is experiencing?
   1. Grieving associated with the potential for death
   2. Powerlessness associated with feelings of being out of control
   3. Fear associated with the perceived threat to biological integrity
   4. Impaired coping associated with inadequate psychological resources

14. A patient who is withdrawn says, "When I have the opportunity, I am going to commit suicide." Which is the **best** response by the nurse?
   1. "You have a lovely family. They need you."
   2. "You must feel overwhelmed to want to kill yourself."
   3. "Let's explore the reasons you have for wanting to live."
   4. "Suicide does not solve problems. Tell me what is wrong."

15. Which situation identified by the nurse reflects the defense mechanism of displacement?
   1. A woman is very nice to her mother-in-law whom she secretly dislikes.
   2. A man says that he is not so bad, so don't believe what they say about him.
   3. An adolescent puts a poor grade on a test out of her mind when at her after-school job.
   4. An older man gets angry with friends after family members attempt to talk with him about his illness.

16. Which is the **best** way for the nurse to support patients' self-esteem needs across the life span?
    1. Employing a positive mental attitude
    2. Providing a nonjudgmental environment
    3. Encouraging social interaction with others
    4. Supporting the use of defense mechanisms

17. A nurse identifies that a patient is mildly anxious. Which assessment of the patient supports this conclusion?
    1. Preoccupied
    2. Forgetful
    3. Fearful
    4. Alert

18. A patient expresses a sense of hopelessness. Which concern identified by the nurse is the priority?
    1. Risk for self-harm
    2. Inability to cope
    3. Powerlessness
    4. Fatigue

19. When assessing a patient for anxiety, which characteristic about anxiety should the nurse consider?
    1. It is triggered by a known stressor.
    2. It occurs simultaneously with fear.
    3. It is a response that is avoidable.
    4. It is a universal experience.

20. A woman with diabetes does not follow her prescribed diet and states, "Everyone with diabetes cheats on their diet." Which defense mechanism does the nurse identify this patient is using?
    1. Rationalization
    2. Sublimation
    3. Undoing
    4. Denial

21. A nurse is interviewing a patient who is a devout Jehovah's Witness. Which nursing statement reflects ethnocentrism?
    1. "Tell me more about your food preferences."
    2. "One of your options is that you can have a kidney transplant."
    3. "You should have a blood transfusion because it is the best way to treat your anemia."
    4. "There is birth control available since you have said you do not want to get pregnant."

22. A neonate is born with a life-threatening anomaly to parents who are Roman Catholic. The primary health-care provider discusses the need for immediate surgery with the parents and they sign an Informed Consent. Which should a culturally competent nurse say to the parents?
    1. "Shall I call a priest so that your baby can receive the Sacrament of the Anointing of the Sick?"
    2. "I will take you to the chapel so that you can pray for your baby during the surgery."
    3. "I will arrange for a Eucharistic minister to give your baby Holy Communion."
    4. "Would you like a nurse who is Roman Catholic to baptize your baby?"

23. A female patient of Arab descent is admitted to the hospital for emergency surgery for an injury sustained in an automobile collision. Considering the Arab culture, which person will be making health-care decisions?
1. The matriarch of the family
2. The woman's oldest son
3. The patient's husband
4. The patient

24. A 4-year-old boy is admitted to the emergency department and diagnosed with leukemia. The parents are informed that their child has an excellent prognosis if treated with chemotherapy. The parents are practicing Christian Scientists and adamantly refuse drug therapy. Which should the nurse do?
1. Encourage the parents to seek the prayers of one of the church's practitioners.
2. Explain to the parents how the chemotherapeutic regimen will cure the leukemia.
3. Talk with the nursing supervisor about referring this situation to the ethics committee.
4. Accept the decision based on the first amendment of the Constitution of the United States.

25. A home care nurse provides nursing services for a community of people who practice the Amish religion and follow a simple lifestyle. Which statement is **unrelated** to the beliefs and values of Amish people?
1. "I am going to have my baby at home rather than in a hospital."
2. "I need permission from my church before I can have surgery."
3. "Please find a nursing home for my father who has dementia."
4. "I do not want anything done to me to prolong my life."

26. A nurse is caring for a patient who is Native American. Which is essential for the nurse to do to provide culturally competent nursing care that is **unique** to Native Americans?
1. Treat the body of a deceased person with respect.
2. Limit access to the patient to just immediate family members.
3. Support hot and cold remedies as long as they do not harm the patient.
4. Provide privacy when family members perform rituals that involve chanting.

27. A primary health-care provider orders a regular diet for a patient of the Jewish faith who follows a kosher diet. Which meals arranged by the nurse are culturally appropriate? **Select all that apply.**
1. _____Chicken lo main, fried rice, pineapple chunks, and tea
2. _____Sliced beef, mixed vegetables, baked potato, and cola
3. _____Hamburger on a bun, potato chips, and milk
4. _____Curried shrimp, egg noodles, and coffee
5. _____Eggs, buttered roll, and orange juice
6. _____Oatmeal, toast, and hot chocolate

28. A family from Asia immigrates to the United States. Which of the following reflect the concept of acculturation? **Select all that apply.**
1. _____Family members take several herbs daily.
2. _____Husband is attending school to learn English.
3. _____Wife prepared a meal with turkey on Thanksgiving.
4. _____Grandparents live in the same house as the rest of the family.
5. _____The children demonstrate respect for their parents and grandparents.

29. A nurse must provide culturally competent nursing care to a patient. Place the following in the order in which they should be performed.
1. Provide care that incorporates the patient's specific beliefs, values, and health-care practices.
2. Recall the beliefs, values, and health-care practices associated with the patient's culture.
3. Explore the patient's specific beliefs, values, and health-care practices.
4. Explore own beliefs, values, and health-care practices.

Answer: _____________

30. A nurse is caring for a woman who is hospitalized because of severe burns to the right hand as a result of a stove-top fire. The patient follows Hinduism. Which should the nurse do to meet the patient's spiritual/cultural needs? **Select all that apply.**
1. _____Provide privacy when the husband visits the patient.
2. _____Assign a nursing assistant to assist the patient with meals.
3. _____Recognize that pain may be stoically accepted by the patient.
4. _____Ensure that a female nurse aid helps the patient with hygienic practices.
5. _____Give her sacred gold necklace to her husband to be taken home for safe-keeping.

31. A nurse is caring for a patient who is a member of the Church of Jesus Christ of Latter-day Saints. Which questions by the nurse are culturally sensitive? **Select all that apply.**
1. _____"Which is the best way for me to care for your sacred undergarment while you are in surgery?"
2. _____"Shall I call a priest to bring you the Eucharist in the morning before your surgery?"
3. _____"Would you like orange juice to be included with your breakfast?"
4. _____"Do you want me to place the head of your bed toward Mecca?"
5. _____"Should I tell the dietitian that you want a vegetarian diet?"

32. A woman who is a member of the Seventh-day Adventist Church is pregnant and considering an abortion. According to her religious beliefs, in which circumstances can this woman decide to have an abortion? **Select all that apply.**
1. _____Form of birth control
2. _____Mother's life is in jeopardy
3. _____Gender selection of the fetus
4. _____Pregnancy resulted from rape
5. _____Congenital anomaly in the fetus

33. A male patient with Latino heritage is diagnosed with hypertension. The nurse reviews the primary health-care provider's orders, obtains the patient's vital signs, and interviews the patient and patient's wife. Which should the nurse do?
1. Obtain the patient's vital signs again in one hour.
2. Explain to the wife that garlic will not help lower her husband's blood pressure.
3. Explore with the couple the fact that prayer will not lower a person's blood pressure.
4. Accept the couple's decision about consuming a clove of garlic and the juice of a lemon daily.

PATIENT'S CLINICAL RECORD

Primary Health-Care Provider's Orders
2-gram sodium diet
Vital signs every 4 hours
Hydrochlorothiazide (HCTZ) 25 mg by mouth once a day
Furosemide 20 mg by mouth once a day

Patient's Vital Signs
Temperature: 98.8°F, orally
Pulse: 88 beats per minute, bounding
Respirations: 22 breaths per minute, unlabored
Blood pressure: 160/94 mm Hg

Patient and Spouse Interview
Patient: "I am going to pray because God has kept me healthy up to now."
Patient's Wife: "We decided that my husband will eat a clove of garlic and drink the juice from a lemon every day."

34. When the nurse analyzes a patient's statements, which statements **best** reflect the dimension of self-esteem? **Select all that apply.**
1. _____"I really like the me that I see."
2. _____"What do I want to achieve?"
3. _____"How do I appear to others?"
4. _____"I like things my way."
5. _____"I'm OK, you're OK."

35. Anxiety can progress through levels of severity from mild to panic. The patient's level of anxiety will influence how the nurse approaches the patient situation. Place these patient statements in order as anxiety progresses from mild, to moderate, to severe, and finally to panic.
1. "I want to know more about the surgery I am having tomorrow."
2. "I don't think I am going to make it through the surgery tomorrow."
3. "I can't concentrate and all I think about is the pain I may have tomorrow."
4. "I get butterflies in my stomach when I think about the surgery tomorrow."

Answer: ____________________

36. A nurse is caring for a patient with a comprehension deficit. Which should the nurse do to **best** support this patient? **Select all that apply.**
1. _____Ask that unclear words be repeated.
2. _____Speak directly in front of the patient.
3. _____Make a referral for a hearing evaluation.
4. _____Establish structured activities of daily living.
5. _____Paraphrase statements when they are not understood.

37. Which nursing actions demonstrate support of human dignity in the practice of nursing? **Select all that apply.**
1. _____Maintaining confidentiality of information about patients
2. _____Supporting the rights of others to refuse treatment
3. _____Obtaining sufficient data to make inferences
4. _____Calling patients by their preferred name
5. _____Staying at the scene of an accident

38. A preoperative patient is anxious about pending elective surgery. Which are the **best** ways for the nurse to help the patient reduce the anxiety? **Select all that apply.**
1. _____Involve significant others.
2. _____Use distraction techniques.
3. _____Explore identified concerns.
4. _____Foster verbalization of feelings.
5. _____Use progressive desensitization strategies.

39. Which might a patient be at risk for in the psychosocial domain when the nursing assessment indicates that the patient is almost completely paralyzed? **Select all that apply.**
1. _____Infection
2. _____Self-harm
3. _____Constipation
4. _____Hopelessness
5. _____Powerlessness

40. A dying patient is withdrawn and depressed. Which nursing actions are therapeutic? **Select all that apply.**
1. _____Assisting the patient to focus on positive thoughts daily
2. _____Explaining that the patient should focus on future goals
3. _____Remaining available in case the patient wants to talk
4. _____Accepting the patient's behavioral adaptation
5. _____Offering the patient advice when appropriate

PSYCHOLOGICAL SUPPORT: ANSWERS AND RATIONALES

1. 1. Although a back rub may provide physical comfort, at this time the patient requires psychosocial comfort. Offering to provide a back rub changes the subject and may cut off further communication.
2. Sitting quietly by the patient's bedside conveys nonjudgmental acceptance of the statement and provides emotional support. Silence may precipitate further communication.
3. Telling the family about the patient's statement is a violation of confidentiality.
4. This is not an appropriate time to initiate an intellectual discussion. The patient's needs are in the psychosocial domain (affective domain).

2. 1. This scenario is an example of denial. Denial is being used when a person ignores or refuses to acknowledge something unacceptable or unpleasant.
2. This scenario is not an example of repression. Repression is an unconscious mechanism whereby painful or unpleasant ideas are kept from conscious awareness.
3. This scenario is not an example of introjection. Introjection is the taking into one's personality the norms and values of another as a means of reducing anxiety.
4. This scenario is not an example of dissociation. Dissociation occurs when a person segregates a group of thoughts from consciousness or when an object or idea is segregated from its emotional significance in an effort to avoid emotional distress.

3. 1. Panic attacks cannot be prevented if identified early, and they do not have a slow onset. Panic attacks usually occur suddenly and spontaneously, build to a peak in 10 minutes or less, and last from several minutes to as long as an hour.
2. People can experience anxiety along a continuum from no anxiety to mild, moderate, severe, or panic, just as health is viewed along a continuum from illness to health.
3. Healthy people experience anxiety when physically or emotionally threatened. Anxiety is a universal response to a threat. People will feel anxious when exposed to something new that is a threat to self-identity or self-esteem.
4. A realistic danger triggers fear, not anxiety.

4. 1. Trust is not the nurse's perceiving the patient's emotions accurately. Trust is established when a patient has confidence in the nurse because the nurse demonstrates competence and respect for the patient and behaves in a predictable way.
2. Empathy is the nurse's ability to have insight into the feelings, emotions, and behavior of the patient.
3. Sympathy is more than expressing concern and sorrow for a patient but also contains an element of pity. When sympathetic, the nurse may let personal feelings interfere with the therapeutic relationship, which can impair judgment and limit the ability to identify realistic solutions to problems. Although sympathy is a caring response, it is not therapeutic, as is empathy.
4. Autonomy is being self-directed, not being able to perceive another person's emotions.

5. 1. Defense mechanisms are used to reduce anxiety and achieve or maintain emotional balance. If a nurse identifies reality and does not recognize the patient's need to use defense mechanisms, the patient will become more anxious, even to the point of panic.
2. Denying the use of a defense mechanism usually does not precipitate withdrawal. Behavioral responses usually include irritability, increased motor activity, and even anger.
3. Denying a patient the use of a defense mechanism will contribute to ineffective coping, not facilitate effective coping.
4. Denying the use of a defense mechanism will not encourage emotional growth. Emotional growth develops as a result of gaining insight into behavior, recognizing reality, and addressing problems constructively.

6. 1. This scenario is an example of intellectualization. Intellectualization is the use of reasoning to avoid facing unacceptable stimuli in an effort to protect the self from anxiety.
2. This scenario is not an example of introjection. Introjection is the taking into one's personality the norms and values of another as a means of reducing anxiety.

3. This scenario is not an example of depression. Depression is not a defense mechanism; it is an altered mood indicated by feelings of sadness, discouragement, and loss of interest in usual pleasurable activities.
4. This scenario is not an example of denial. Denial is ignoring or refusing to acknowledge something unacceptable or unpleasant.

7. 1. During mild anxiety, the pulse, respirations, and blood pressure remain at the resting rate.
2. During moderate anxiety, the pulse, respirations, and blood pressure are slightly elevated in response to the stimulation of the autonomic nervous system.
3. During severe anxiety, the pulse, respirations, and blood pressure are more than just slightly elevated. The pulse and respirations are rapid and may be irregular, and the blood pressure is high, not just slightly elevated.
4. During a panic attack, the pulse and respirations are very rapid and may be irregular, the blood pressure will be high, and the patient may hyperventilate. If a panic attack is extreme, the blood pressure may suddenly drop and cause fainting.

8. 1. This scenario is not an example of compensation. Compensation is making an attempt to achieve respect in one area as a substitute for a weakness in another area.
2. This scenario not an example of minimization. Minimization is not admitting to the significance of one's own behavior, thereby reducing one's responsibility.
3. This scenario is an example of repression. Repression is an unconscious mechanism in which painful or unpleasant ideas are kept from conscious awareness.
4. This scenario is not an example of regression. Regression is resorting to an earlier, more comfortable pattern of behavior that was successful in earlier years but is now inappropriate.

9. 1. Patients generally follow hospital policies because they recognize that they are designed to keep patients safe. When they do not follow rules, usually it is for a reason other than because they are angry.
2. Patients have an opportunity to choose foods they like from the menu, to request alternative meals if they are unhappy with the food that arrives, and to ask family members to bring in food as long as the food is permitted on the ordered diet.
3. All behavior has meaning. Acting-out behaviors that reflect attempts to control events often are covert expressions of feeling powerless.
4. Most hospital units have a lounge that supports patients' needs to have a change of scenery from their rooms.

10. 1. Exercise stimulates endorphin production, which promotes a sense of well-being and euphoria. Also, endorphins act as opiates and produce analgesia by modulating the transmission of pain perception.
2. Exercise improves, not interferes with, one's ability to concentrate and solve problems by increasing circulation, which facilitates oxygenation of brain cells.
3. Exercise promotes, not reduces, metabolism of epinephrine, thereby minimizing autonomic arousal and decreasing vigilance associated with the anxious response.
4. The acidity of blood is increased, not decreased, by exercise. This improves digestion and metabolism and thereby increases one's energy level.

11. 1. Touching the patient conveys concern and caring and is supportive. Quiet support provides a nonjudgmental environment in which the patient is allowed to cry, which is the expression of a feeling.
2. Leaving abandons the patient at a time when the patient needs emotional support.
3. Conveying this information to the patient's family is a violation of confidentiality.
4. Exploring the patient's feelings is premature. The patient requires time to cry as a way to express sad feelings.

12. 1. This scenario is not an example of rationalization. Rationalization is used to justify in some socially acceptable way ideas, feelings, or behavior through explanations that appear to be logical.
2. This scenario is not an example of minimization. Minimization is not admitting to the significance of one's own behavior, thereby reducing one's responsibility.

3. This scenario is not an example of substitution. Substitution is replacement of an unattainable, unavailable, or unacceptable goal, emotion, or motive with one that is attainable, available, or acceptable in an effort to reduce anxiety, frustration or disappointment.
4. **This scenario is an example of projection. Projection is attributing thoughts, emotions, motives, or characteristics within oneself to others.**

13. 1. A characteristic of grieving is that the person must express distress regarding a loss or potential loss. This patient is asking questions, not displaying distress related to a perceived impending death.
2. This statement does not reflect powerlessness. People who are powerless usually do not ask questions.
3. **This statement supports the fact that the patient is experiencing fear. A characteristic of fear is the verbalization of feelings of apprehension and alarm related to an identifiable source.**
4. This statement does not indicate that the patient is coping ineffectively or has inadequate psychological resources. The patient is gathering data by appropriately asking questions, which is an effective, task-oriented action in the coping process.

14. 1. This statement is inappropriate; the patient is unable to cope, is selecting the ultimate escape, and is not capable of meeting the needs of others; this response also may precipitate feelings such as guilt.
2. **This statement identifies feelings and invites further communication; it uses the interviewing technique of reflection.**
3. This denies the patient's feelings; the patient must focus on the negatives before exploring the positives.
4. This is a judgmental response that may cut off communication. This response is too direct, and the patient may not consciously know what is wrong.

15. 1. This scenario is an example of reaction formation, not displacement. Reaction formation is when a person develops conscious attitudes, behaviors, interests, and feelings that are the exact opposite to unconscious attitudes, interests, and feelings.
2. This scenario is an example of minimization. Minimization allows a person to decrease responsibility for one's own behavior.
3. This scenario is an example of suppression, not displacement. Suppression is a conscious attempt to put unpleasant thoughts out of the conscious mind to be dealt with at a later time.
4. **This scenario is an example of displacement. Displacement is the transfer of emotion from one person or object to a person or an object that is more acceptable and less threatening.**

16. 1. The nurse's personal attitudes should not be imposed on the patient. An attitude is a mental position or feeling toward a person, an object, or an idea.
2. **When the nurse establishes a nonjudgmental environment and functions without biases, preconceptions, or stereotypes and avoids challenging a patient's values and beliefs, a patient's self-esteem is supported.**
3. This may or may not support self-esteem needs. The benefit of this intervention depends on the relationships that develop and whether they promote self-worth.
4. The support of a defense mechanism results in reality distortion. The use of defense mechanisms should be accepted, not supported. The nurse just should recognize when defense mechanisms are being used because all behavior has meaning.

17. 1. Preoccupation reflects moderate, not mild, anxiety. People with moderate anxiety tend to focus on one issue and use selective attention.
2. Forgetfulness reflects moderate, not mild, anxiety. With mild anxiety, the person increases arousal and perceptual fields and is motivated to learn. With moderate anxiety, the person has a narrowed focus of attention and may become forgetful because of an inability to focus attention.
3. Fearfulness is not a response to anxiety. Fearfulness is a response to an identifiable source, whereas anxiety is caused by an unidentifiable source.
4. **Increased alertness occurs when one is mildly anxious. Alertness and vigilance are the result of an increase in one's**

perceptual field and state of arousal in response to the stimulation of the autonomic nervous system when one feels threatened.

18. **1. Risk for self-harm takes priority over the other three concerns because of the potential for suicide.**
2. Although a person who expresses hopelessness may also demonstrate an inability to manage stressors because of inadequate physical, psychological, behavioral, or cognitive resources, another option identifies a concern that has a higher priority.
3. Although a person who expresses hopelessness may also perceive a lack of personal control over events or situations, another option identifies a concern that has a higher priority.
4. Although a person who expresses hopelessness may also experience an overwhelming sense of exhaustion unrelieved by rest, another option identifies a concern that has a higher priority.

19. 1. Anxiety is triggered by an unknown, not known, stressor.
2. Anxiety and fear do not occur simultaneously. Anxiety is precipitated by an unknown stressor, while fear is precipitated by a known stressor.
3. Anxiety cannot be avoided. It is an expected aspect of everyday living. Every time someone experiences something new, it is a threat to the identity or self-esteem; therefore, people feel anxious.
4. Anxiety is a common and universal response to a threat. Every time people experience something new that is a threat to the identity or self-esteem, they may feel anxious. Anxiety is a psychosocial response to an unknown stress; it may be a vague sense of apprehension at one extreme to impending doom at the other extreme.

20. **1. This is an example of rationalization. Rationalization is used to justify in some socially acceptable way ideas, feelings, or behavior through explanations that appear to be logical.**
2. This is not an example of sublimation. Sublimation is the channeling of primitive sexual or aggressive drives into activities or behaviors that are more socially acceptable, such as sports or creative work.
3. This is not an example of undoing. Undoing is use of actions or words in an attempt to cancel unacceptable thoughts, impulses, or acts. This reduces feelings of guilt through atonement or retribution.
4. This is not an example of denial. Denial is an unconscious protective response that involves a person's ignoring or refusing to acknowledge something unacceptable or unpleasant to reduce anxiety.

21. 1. This statement reflects culturally sensitive, appropriate, and competent nursing care. The nurse is collecting information to individualize nursing care.
2. This statement does not impose the nurse's values, beliefs, and practices onto the patient (cultural imposition) because it is just providing the patient with an additional option; however, it is culturally insensitive. A person who is a devout Jehovah's Witness does not believe in organ transplantation, abortion, or sterilization. Jehovah's Witnesses do allow birth control, autopsy, and cremation.
3. This is an example of ethnocentrism. Ethnocentrism is viewing one's own values, beliefs, and practices as being superior or more acceptable or best in comparison to the patient's values, beliefs, and practices. A person who is a devout Jehovah's Witness does not believe in the use of blood or blood products even in a life-threatening situation. Jehovah's Witnesses do believe in the use of artificial blood expanders.
4. This statement does not reflect ethnocentrism. The patient has stated a need and the nurse is providing information regarding how to meet that need.

22. 1. The infant should be baptized before receiving the Sacrament of the Anointing of the Sick.
2. This is presumptuous, inappropriate, and authoritative. The parents may not have the energy, focus, or desire to pray.
3. Individuals must be baptized before they can receive Holy Communion. Holy Communion usually is administered after studying the scriptures and basics of the Roman Catholic religion and reaching the age of reason (usually 7 years of age). Nothing should be put into the mouth of an individual being prepared for surgery, to prevent aspiration.

4. **A member of the Roman Catholic faith can baptize in an emergency if a priest is unavailable. The surgery is imminent.**

23. 1. Women are not the decision makers in families of Arab heritage regardless of their age or status.
 2. This is not the role of the oldest son while the patient's husband is still alive.
 3. **In Arab heritage, women do not make autonomous health-care decisions; husbands are the decision makers for their wives.**
 4. Women are not the decision makers in families of Arab heritage.

24. 1. While prayer can be powerful, it alone will not cure leukemia. Church practitioners are trained by the church to pray for members. Church members believe that physical illness and sin are states of mind, correctable through properly applied prayer.
 2. This is an inappropriate intervention at this time. The parents are steadfastly and obstinately refusing drug therapy. It also provides false reassurance because not all children with leukemia experience a cure after undergoing chemotherapy.
 3. **This is an ethical dilemma. An ethics committee is an advisory body with a multidisciplinary composition that facilitates the exploration and resolution of ethical issues that occur within the facility.**
 4. The United States court system can intervene on the behalf of infants and children when parents refuse life-saving treatments. The nurse is not being an advocate for the child in this situation.

25. 1. Amish people believe that birth and death are phases of life and should occur in the home.
 2. Amish people need permission from their church before receiving care in a hospital. They accept anesthesia, surgery, blood transfusions, blood products, dental care, and organ transplants other than the heart (the heart is considered the soul of the body).
 3. **It is unlikely that an Amish person would place a family member in a nursing home. Amish people believe in caring for ill family members in their home and prefer to die in the home with family members by the bedside. They have a strong commitment to family members and members of the community.**
 4. Amish people believe that end of life care be limited so that assets are used for the living.

26. 1. Everyone, dead or alive, should be treated with respect at all times.
 2. Native Americans believe illness is a concern of the family, extended family, and tribe. The nurse should support visits from those people who are desired by the patient.
 3. People with Hispanic and Latino heritage, not Native Americans, believe in the use of "hot" and "cold" remedies to heal illnesses.
 4. **Native Americans engage in rituals, ceremonies, and exorcisms that may involve chanting, dancing, and the wearing of amulets. Privacy should be provided.**

27. 1. **All the foods and fluid in this meal are permitted on a kosher diet. Meat from animals that are cloven footed, cud chewing, and slaughtered and prepared following strict laws of Kashrut (kosher diet) are permitted.**
 2. **All of the foods and fluid in this meal are permitted together on a kosher diet. Beef is from a cow, a cud-chewing animal, which is permitted on a kosher diet as long as it is not served at the same meal as a dairy product.**
 3. Hamburger is ground beef and milk is a dairy product. Meat and dairy products cannot be served at the same meal. Each requires separate sets of dishes, pots, pans, and utensils to ensure that they remain separate and do not contaminate each other. Potato chips are permitted with meals that contain meat or dairy products.
 4. Only fish that have scales and fins are permitted on a kosher diet. Shellfish such as shrimp, crab, and lobster are not permitted on a kosher diet.
 5. **All of the foods and this fluid in this meal are permitted together on a kosher diet. This meal does not contain both dairy and meat products and does not contain pork.**
 6. **All these foods and fluid are permitted at the same meal when a person is following a kosher diet. This meal does not contain both dairy and meat products and does not contain pork.**

28. 1. This is not an example of acculturation. Asian cultures have a rich history of Eastern medicine including the use of herbs, applications of hot and cold, and acupuncture to reestablish balance within the body.

2. Acculturation is the process of adapting to a new environment or situation that is different from one's own. Currently, the dominant language in the United States is English. The husband is attempting to adapt to the United States.

3. Eating turkey on Thanksgiving is a tradition in the United States. The wife's making a turkey on Thanksgiving is incorporating a tradition associated with their new country into the family's practices.

4. This is not an example of acculturation. Several generations of family members living in the same household is an accepted practice within an Asian family, not something that generally is practiced in the United States. However, this may become more prevalent in the United States as the economy continues to decline and young adults and retired individuals do not have the economic resources to maintain a separate home.

5. This does not necessarily reflect acculturation. Individuals from Asian cultures value respect for elders and are subordinate to authority. This may or may not reflect the attitude of all individuals living in the United States. Some believe older adults no longer have the same value as when they were younger because they do not contribute to society.

29. 4. A nurse must know herself or himself before caring for others. Personal values, beliefs, practices, biases, and prejudices must be identified to ensure that they are not imposed on patients.

2. Often there are commonalities in the values, beliefs, and practices within a culture. It is important for the nurse to be aware of these commonalities to promote culturally competent nursing care.

3. Individuals within a culture do not always ascribe to the beliefs, values, and practices of the collective culture. Preferences must be explored with patients to ensure that nursing care is individualized.

1. Knowing about the beliefs, values, and practices within a culture and specific to an individual is not enough. A nurse must respect and provide care that adheres to the beliefs, values, and practices of each individual to provide culturally appropriate and competent nursing care.

30. 1. Public displays of affection are prohibited. Touching, hugging, and kissing are considered strictly private matters.

2. Individuals who practice Hinduism eat with only the right hand because the left hand is used for toileting activities.

3. Followers of Hinduism believe that pain is caused by the anger of a higher power and therefore one must bear the condition and situation.

4. Women are modest and prefer female direct patient caregivers. Patient privacy is a priority.

5. Wearing a sacred gold necklace should be permitted. It can be removed only with consent from the patient when it will interfere with a necessary procedure.

31. 1. This question is culturally sensitive. The sacred undergarment worn by a member of the Church of Jesus Christ of Latter-day Saints is removed only for bathing. It can be removed for surgery but must be treated with respect.

2. This question is culturally insensitive. Receiving the Eucharist (Holy Communion) is a practice of religions such as Roman Catholic and Episcopalian.

3. This question is culturally sensitive. Dietary practices prohibit the intake of coffee and tea, not orange juice.

4. This question is culturally insensitive. Positioning the head of the bed toward Mecca meets the spiritual needs of those who follow the Islamic faith.

5. This question is culturally insensitive. Members of the Church of Jesus Christ of Latter-day Saints are permitted to eat a moderate amount of meat.

32. 1. The Seventh-day Adventist Church, a Protestant denomination, opposes abortion for convenience. Abortion as a form of birth control is unacceptable.

2. The Seventh-day Adventist Church, a Protestant denomination, permits abortion in extreme situations such as when the life of the mother is in

jeopardy. The life of the mother becomes the priority.

3. The Seventh-day Adventist Church, a Protestant denomination, does not condone abortion as an intervention of convenience. Abortion to prevent the birth of an infant with an undesirable gender is not condoned.
4. **The Seventh-day Adventist Church, a Protestant denomination, permits abortion in extreme situations such as when the pregnancy resulted from rape or incest.**
5. **The Seventh-day Adventist Church, a Protestant denomination, permits abortion in extreme situations such as when a fetus has a severe congenital anomaly.**

33. 1. It is unnecessary to obtain the patient's vital signs in one hour. Although the blood pressure is increased, it is not at a dangerous level. The primary health-care provider ordered that vital signs be obtained every 4 hours.
2. Garlic has hypolipemic and antiplatelet properties that can help lower blood pressure.
3. Prayer, meditation, and biofeedback exercises can help lower the vital signs, especially heart rate and blood pressure.
4. **Latino and Hispanic individuals believe illness is caused by an imbalance in hot and cold principles. Hypertension is considered a "hot" illness and therefore should be treated with "cold" therapies. Cold therapies include the ingestion of foods such as citrus fruits, garlic, and bananas.**

34. 1. **This statement best reflects the dimension of self-esteem. Self-esteem is a person's self-evaluation of one's own worth or value. A person whose self-concept comes close to one's ideal self generally will have a high self-esteem.**
2. This statement reflects one's self-expectations, not self-esteem. Establishing expectations contributes to the composition of the ideal self.
3. This statement reflects self-concept, not self-esteem. Self-concept is an individual's knowledge about oneself. Self-concept is derived from all the collective beliefs and images about oneself as a result of interaction with the environment, society, and feedback from others.
4. This statement is a reflection of a patient's need to be autonomous and self-reliant. Having confidence in one's ability to complete a task is only one component of self-concept.
5. **This statement reflects the dimension of self-esteem. By stating "I'm OK," the person demonstrates self-acceptance.**

35. 1. **Mild anxiety is a slightly aroused state that enhances perception, learning, and performance of activities.**
4. **Moderate anxiety increases the arousal state that precipitates feelings of tension and nervousness. The heart and respiratory rates increase, and the person may have mild gastrointestinal symptoms, such as a feeling of butterflies in the stomach.**
3. **Severe anxiety consumes the person's physical and emotional energy. Perceptions are decreased, and the person focuses on limited aspects of what is precipitating the anxiety.**
2. **Panic is an overwhelming state where the person feels out of control. Perceptions may be distorted and exaggerated, and the person may have feelings of impending doom.**

36. 1. **To best support a patient the nurse must understand what the patient is communicating. When a patient's message is unclear the nurse must obtain clarification.**
2. This action does not facilitate comprehension. It helps a patient with a hearing deficit recognize that someone is speaking, and it facilitates lip reading if the patient has the ability to read lips.
3. The patient's problem is a decreased ability to process and understand information, not a hearing loss.
4. **New experiences require a person to process information and problem solve, which is difficult to do for the person with a comprehension deficit. Lack of understanding is threatening to feelings of safety and security. Structure and routines provide predictability, which limits confusion, disorientation, and anxiety.**
5. **Paraphrasing a message uses different words that the patient may understand, promoting decoding of the message and communication.**

37. 1. **Confidentiality respects the patient's right to privacy, which is a component of human dignity.**

2. This supports the right of a patient to self-determination, which is based on the concept of freedom, not human dignity.

3. This reflects the nurse's attempt to seek the truth, not support human dignity.

4. **Calling patients by their given name demonstrates respect for the individual. Avoid names such as "dear," "sweetie," "honey," and "grandma," or "grandpa," because they are demeaning and disrespectful.**

5. This reflects a nurse's attempt to be responsible and accountable, not support human dignity.

38. 1. Significant others generally are as anxious as the patient because anxiety is contagious. Anxious significant others bring to the discussion their own emotional problems that can misdirect the focus from the patient as well as compound the problem.

2. Although distraction techniques, such as guided imagery, can help manage stress, other options offer a more effective interventions to reduce anxiety.

3. **Exploring identified concerns individualizes the nurse's interventions. Specific issues can be addressed and knowledge deficits corrected.**

4. **Using interviewing techniques encourages the patient to verbalize feelings and explore concerns, which reduce anxiety. Verbalization uses energy, makes concerns recognizable, and promotes problem solving.**

5. Anxiety is not something one can desensitize oneself to by increasing exposure to the stressor. With anxiety, the stressor is unknown.

39. 1. The risk for infection is a concern in the physiological, not the psychosocial, domain.

2. Data do not support the concern that the patient will cause self-harm. The data related to the risk for self-harm are an expression of a desire to harm oneself, commit suicide, or die.

3. The risk for constipation is a concern in the physiological, not the psychosocial, domain.

4. **A person who feels hopeless sees no solution to the problem. A person who is almost completely paralyzed may not be able to mobilize energy on his or her own behalf to move forward and achieve goals.**

5. **People who are unable to care for themselves independently often perceive a lack of control over events. The nurse should be alert to the presence of data that support powerlessness.**

40. 1. Focusing on positive thoughts is inappropriate because it denies the patient's feelings; the patient needs to focus on the future loss.

2. Focusing on future goals is inappropriate because it denies the patient's feelings; the patient needs to focus on the impending death. The nurse should not be telling the patient what should be the focus of care.

3. **Remaining available to the patient indicates that the nurse is not abandoning the patient. The nurse's presence provides quiet support without intruding on the patient's coping.**

4. **Depression is the fourth stage of grieving according to Kübler-Ross; patients become withdrawn and noncommunicative when feeling a loss of control and recognizing future losses. The nurse should accept the behavior and be available if the patient wants to verbalize feelings.**

5. It is never appropriate to offer advice; people must explore their alternatives and come to their own conclusions.

Teaching and Learning

KEYWORDS

The following words include nursing/medical terminology, concepts, principles, and information relevant to content specifically addressed in the chapter or associated with topics presented in it. English dictionaries, nursing textbooks, and medical dictionaries, such as *Taber's Cyclopedic Medical Dictionary,* are resources that can be used to expand your knowledge and understanding of these words and related information.

Behavior modification
Continuing education program
Feedback
Focus group
Inservice education program
Learning domains:
  Affective:
    Receiving
    Responding
    Valuing
    Organizing
    Characterizing
  Cognitive:
    Acquisition
    Comprehension
    Application
    Analysis
    Synthesis
    Evaluation
  Psychomotor:
    Set
    Guided response
    Mechanism
    Complex overt response
    Adaptation
    Origination
Locus of control:
  External
  Internal
Motivation
Orientation program
Pre-test, post-test
Readiness
Reading level
Reinforcement
Teaching:
  Formal
  Informal
Teaching methods:
  Active learning
  Audiovisual aids
  Case study
  Computer-assisted instruction
  Demonstration
  Discussion
  Lecture
  Programmed instruction
  Return demonstration
  Role-playing
  Simulation
  Written material

TEACHING AND LEARNING: QUESTIONS

1. A nurse is caring for a patient who has type 1 diabetes and an ulcer on the big toe of the right foot. The nurse plans to review how to perform self-blood glucose monitoring, self-administer an injection, and apply a sterile dressing to the ulcer on the toe. The nurse identifies that the patient is a kinesthetic learner. Which teaching strategy is **most** appropriate for the nurse to use with this patient?
1. Give verbal instructions and encourage a discussion
2. Provide occasions to touch and handle equipment
3. Present pictures and illustrations
4. Use models and videos

2. A nurse is assessing a patient to determine educational needs. Which is **most** important for the nurse to consider?
   1. Make no assumptions about the patient.
   2. Teaching may be informal or formal in nature.
   3. The teaching plan should be documented on appropriate records.
   4. A copy of the teaching-learning contract should be given to the patient.

3. Which is the **primary** reason why nurses attend continuing education programs?
   1. Update professional knowledge.
   2. Network within the nursing profession.
   3. Fulfill requirements for an advanced degree.
   4. Graduate from an accredited nursing program.

4. A nurse is designing a teaching-learning program for a patient who is to be discharged from the hospital. After developing a nurse-patient relationship, which should the nurse do **next?**
   1. Identify the patient's locus of control.
   2. Use a variety of teaching methods appropriate for the patient.
   3. Formulate an achievable, measurable, and realistic patient goal.
   4. Assess the patient's current understanding of the content to be taught.

5. A nurse is teaching an older adult how to perform a dressing change. Which nursing action is **most** important to address a developmental stress of older adults?
   1. Speak louder when talking to the patient.
   2. Use terminology understandable to the patient.
   3. Have the patient provide a return demonstration.
   4. Allow more time for the patient to process information.

6. A nurse is planning a weight-reduction program with an obese patient. Which should the nurse anticipate will be the **most** important component that will determine the success or failure of this program?
   1. Rewarding compliant behavior with favorite foods
   2. Encouraging at least 1 hour of exercise daily
   3. Using an 800-calorie daily dietary regimen
   4. Setting realistic goals

7. A nurse is teaching a patient recently diagnosed with diabetes mellitus the step-by-step procedure of administering an insulin injection by using an orange. However, after two sessions of practice the patient is still reluctant to self-administer the insulin. Which should the nurse do?
   1. Keep reinforcing the principles that have been presented.
   2. Have the patient administer the injection to an orange again.
   3. Give the patient an opportunity to explore concerns about the injection.
   4. Determine if a member of the family is willing to administer the insulin.

8. Every person who attended a smoking cessation educational program completed a questionnaire. Which is this type of evaluation called?
   1. Survey
   2. Post-test
   3. Case study
   4. Focus group

9. A nurse educator designed various educational programs that employ role-playing as a teaching strategy. Which group of people should the nurse anticipate will benefit the **most** from role-playing?
   1. Older adults preparing to retire from the workforce
   2. Men unwilling to admit that they have a drinking problem
   3. Adolescents learning to abstain from recreational drug use
   4. Middle-aged adults preparing for total-knee replacement surgery

10. To be **most** effective, at which grade reading level should the nurse prepare written educational medical material?
1. Fourth-grade
2. Eighth-grade
3. Tenth-grade
4. Sixth-grade

11. A nurse uses computer-assisted instruction as a strategy when providing preoperative teaching. Which should the nurse explain to preoperative patients is the **greatest** advantage of computer-assisted instruction?
1. Learners can progress at their own rate.
2. It is the least expensive teaching strategy.
3. There are opportunities for pre- and post-testing.
4. Information is presented in a well-organized format.

12. A nurse is teaching a preschool-aged child. Which teaching method is **most** appropriate for the nurse to use when teaching a child in this age group?
1. Demonstrations
2. Coloring books
3. Small groups
4. Videos

13. A nurse is attending a class about a new intravenous pump presented by the hospital staff education department. Which is this type of educational program?
1. Continuing education program
2. Inservice education program
3. Certification program
4. Orientation program

14. A nurse is planning teaching about weight-reduction strategies to an obese patient. Which should the nurse assess **first** before implementing the teaching plan?
1. Intelligence
2. Experience
3. Motivation
4. Strengths

15. A nurse is planning to engage a patient in a program to learn about a newly diagnosed illness. Which psychosocial response to the illness will have the **greatest** impact on the patient's future success of learning?
1. Fear
2. Denial
3. Fatigue
4. Anxiety

16. A nurse must implement a teaching plan for a patient recently diagnosed with heart failure. Which should the nurse do **first**?
1. Identify the patient's level of recognition of the need for learning.
2. Frame the goal within the patient's value system.
3. Determine the patient's preferred learning style.
4. Assess the patient's personal support system.

17. Which of the following teaching-learning concepts that moves from one extreme to the other is basic to all teaching plans?
1. Cognitive to the affective domain
2. Formal to the informal
3. Simple to the complex
4. Broad to the specific

18. A nurse is teaching a postoperative patient deep breathing and coughing exercises. Which method of instruction is **most** appropriate in this situation?
1. Explanation
2. Demonstration
3. Video presentation
4. Brochure with pictures

19. A nurse is teaching a patient colostomy care in relation to the affective domain. Which teaching method is **most** effective for this situation?
1. Discussing a pamphlet about colostomy care from the American Cancer Society
2. Exploring how the patient feels about having a colostomy
3. Providing a demonstration on how to do colostomy care
4. Showing a videotape demonstrating colostomy care

20. A school nurse is teaching a class of adolescents about avoiding smoking and includes role-playing as a creative learning activity. Which is the **primary** reason for using role-playing?
1. Provides more fun than other methods
2. Eliminates the need for media equipment
3. Requires active participation by the learner
4. Gives the learner the opportunity to be another person

21. A culturally competent nurse is planning to teach a patient about a new regimen of self-care. Which must the nurse assess **first** about the patient before implementing the teaching plan?
1. Religious affiliation
2. Support system
3. National origin
4. Health beliefs

22. A nurse is planning to teach the patient how to self-administer a colostomy irrigation. Place the following actions that the nurse should employ in the order in which they should be implemented.
1. Identify the patient's readiness to learn.
2. Involve the patient in learning activities.
3. Identify the patient's motivation to learn.
4. Repeat essential concepts to reinforce learning.
5. Evaluate the patient's learning versus desired outcomes.

Answer: ______________

23. A nursing instructor is evaluating a student nurse's knowledge. Which student behaviors indicate that learning has occurred in the highest level of learning in the cognitive domain? **Select all that apply.**
1. _____Identifies the expected properties of urine
2. _____Explains the importance of producing urine
3. _____Recognizes when something is contaminated
4. _____Compares achieved outcomes with planned outcomes
5. _____Contrasts laboratory results of urine testing against the expected range

24. A nurse is to teach a patient how to change a dressing and irrigate a wound that resulted from the separation of wound edges of an incision and that is healing by secondary intention. The nurse reviews the primary health-care provider's orders, obtains the patient's vital signs, and assesses the patient. Which should the nurse do **next**?
1. Administer the prescribed pain medication and reassess the patient in 30 minutes.
2. Teach the patient how to irrigate the wound and change the dressing.
3. Notify the primary health-care provider of the patient's status.
4. Wait 15 minutes and retake the patient's vital signs.

PATIENT'S CLINICAL RECORD

Primary Health-Care Provider's Orders
Irrigate abdominal wound with 0.9% sodium chloride and apply a wet to damp dressing twice a day.
Oxycodone 7.5 mg every 6 hours prn for incisional pain

Patient's Vital Signs
Temperature: 100.2°F, orally
Pulse: 98 beats per minute
Respirations: 20 breaths per minute
Blood pressure: 140/90 mm Hg

Patient Interview
Patient is quiet and responding with one-phrase answers. States pain is 7 on a scale of 0 to 10. Transferred from chair to bed while bent over and holding abdomen. Patient states, "I can't wait to learn how to do this dressing so that I can go home."

25. A nurse is providing health teaching for a patient with a cognitive deficit. Which interventions by the nurse will support this patient's learning? **Select all that apply.**
1. _____Using simple vocabulary and syntax
2. _____Establishing a structured environment
3. _____Asking that unclear words be repeated
4. _____Speaking directly in front of the patient
5. _____Making a referral for a hearing evaluation

26. A unit secretary tells the nurse that the primary health-care provider has just ordered a low-calorie diet for a patient who is overweight. Place these nursing interventions in the order in which they should be implemented.
1. Verify the dietary order.
2. Determine food preferences.
3. Teach specifics about a low-calorie diet.
4. Review a meal plan designed by the patient.
5. Assess the patient's motivation to follow the diet.

Answer: _______________

27. Which describe a patient with an external locus of control? **Select all that apply.**
1. _____Behaving appropriately to obtain the right to watch a television program
2. _____Is self-motivated when implementing health promotion behaviors
3. _____Wants to please family members with efforts to get well
4. _____Understands the expected outcome of therapy
5. _____Is a self-actualized adult

28. A nurse is teaching a patient with a hearing impairment. Which should the nurse do to facilitate the teaching-learning process? **Select all that apply.**
1. _____Limit educational sessions to 10 minutes.
2. _____Provide information in written format.
3. _____Use at least 2 teaching methods.
4. _____Face the patient when talking.
5. _____Teach in group settings.

29. A nurse formulates teaching goals using action verbs. Which words are examples of verbs employed in learning outcomes in the psychomotor domain? **Select all that apply.**
1. _____Accepts
2. _____Explains
3. _____Performs
4. _____Assembles
5. _____Demonstrates

30. A nurse is assessing the results of dietary teaching for a patient with diabetes mellitus. Which patient behaviors indicate that learning occurred in the affective domain? **Select all that apply.**
   1. _____Discusses which food on the ordered diet must be avoided
   2. _____Eats only food approved on the prescribed special diet
   3. _____Lists foods that are permitted on the diet
   4. _____Asks about which foods can be eaten
   5. _____Avoids food that is high in sugar

31. A community health nurse is caring for a patient who has a pressure ulcer and requires assistance with bathing, grooming, and toileting. Docusate sodium, daily weights, and a dressing change of the wound twice a day are ordered. When performing which nursing interventions should the nurse educate the patient about docusate sodium? **Select all that apply.**
   1. _____Bathing
   2. _____Toileting
   3. _____Daily weights
   4. _____Wound treatment
   5. _____Medication administration

32. After assessing a patient's learning needs, abilities, and motivation and identifying patient goals, the nurse must formulate a teaching plan. Place the following steps in the order in which they should be implemented.
   1. Choose teaching strategies to be employed.
   2. Evaluate the effectiveness of the teaching plan.
   3. Identify the information that the learner must learn.
   4. Organize the information in the sequence that information is to be presented.
   5. Develop instructional materials that will reinforce and supplement information provided in the class.

   Answer: _______________

33. A nurse is planning a teaching plan for an older adult. Which common factors among older adult patients must be considered? **Select all that apply.**
   1. _____Sensory decline occurs as one ages.
   2. _____Learning may require more energy.
   3. _____Intelligence decreases as people age.
   4. _____Older adults rely more on visual rather than auditory learning.
   5. _____Older adult patients are more resistant to change that accompanies new learning.

34. A nurse is teaching a patient who has impaired vision to self-inject insulin. Which should the nurse do to facilitate the teaching-learning process? **Select all that apply.**
   1. _____Obtain an order for automatic-stop syringes.
   2. _____Provide written information in large print.
   3. _____Use audio learning materials.
   4. _____Enunciate each word clearly.
   5. _____Speak slowly.

35. A nurse educator is teaching a class on problem solving and reinforced the concepts of inductive and deductive reasoning using the attached illustration. Which is the **most** important reason why the nurse educator presented this illustration?
   1. It appeals to students who are visual learners.
   2. It employs the concept of positive reinforcement.
   3. It stimulates learning in students with an internal locus of control.
   4. It improves students' conceptual understanding of complex content.

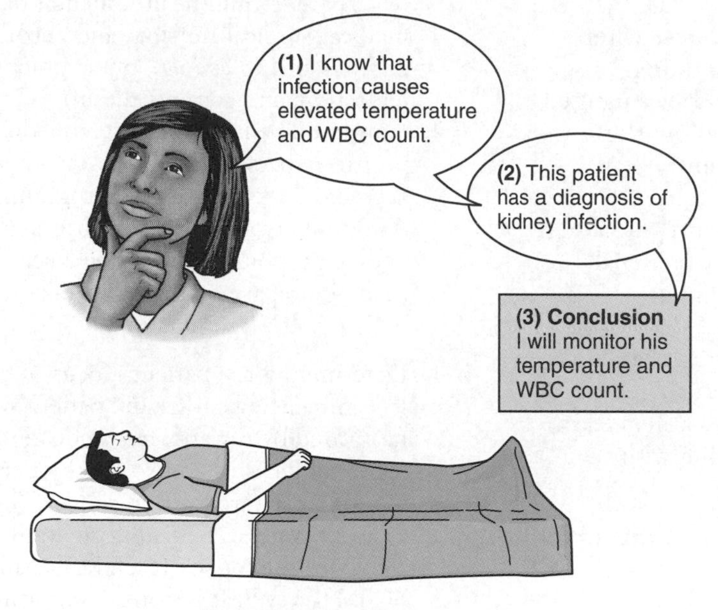

Deductive reasoning

TEACHING AND LEARNING: ANSWERS AND RATIONALES

1. 1. Verbal instructions and discussions are most appropriate to use with patients who are auditory, not kinesthetic, learners. Auditory learners learn best by processing information by listening to words.

2. Kinesthetic learners learn best when processing information by doing. Kinesthetic learners should be engaged in physical activities that allow them to touch and handle equipment.

3. Pictures and illustrations are most appropriate to use with patients who are visual, not kinesthetic, learners. Visual learners learn best by processing information with the eyes.

4. Models and videos are most appropriate to use with patients who are visual, not kinesthetic, learners. Visual learners learn best by processing information with the eyes.

2. 1. Many variables influence an individual's willingness and ability to learn (e.g., readiness, motivation, physical and emotional abilities, education, age, cultural and health beliefs, cognitive abilities). Because everyone is unique with individual needs, the nurse must avoid making assumptions and generalizations.

2. The patient's needs must be identified before teaching formats and strategies are designed.

3. The patient's needs must be identified before the teaching plan is designed, implemented, and documented.

4. The patient's needs must be identified before a plan is designed and a contract is written.

3. 1. Continuing education programs are formal learning experiences designed to update and enhance professional knowledge or skills. This is necessary because of the explosion in information and technology within health care. Some states require evidence of continuing education units (CEUs) for license renewal.

2. Although nurses who attend continuing education programs have the opportunity to network professionally with other nurses, it is not the main purpose of attending a continuing education program.

3. Continuing education programs do not fulfill requirements for an advanced degree. Master's and doctoral programs grant advanced degrees in specialty areas (e.g., parent-child health, mental health, medical-surgical nursing, and gerontology) and practice roles (e.g., nurse practitioner, education, and administration).

4. Continuing education programs do not prepare a person to graduate from an accredited nursing degree program. Associate degree programs, baccalaureate degree programs, and diploma schools of nursing prepare graduates to take the NCLEX-RN examination.

4. 1. Determining the patient's locus of control will influence whether the patient will be motivated by rewards from outside the self (external locus of control) or by personally identified rewards within the self (internal locus of control). This information should influence the nurse's teaching-learning plan. However, it is not the first thing the nurse should do of the options offered.

2. Although a variety of teaching methods should be used so that all the senses are engaged in learning, it is not the first thing the nurse should do of the options offered.

3. Goal setting is accomplished after the nurse gathers essential information that will influence the goal, particularly in relation to the achievable and realistic factors of a goal.

4. Learners bring their own lifetimes of learning to the learning situation. The nurse must customize each teaching plan, capitalize on the patient's previous experience and knowledge, and identify what the patient still needs to know before teaching can begin.

5. 1. Speaking loudly could be demeaning. A normal volume of speaking is appropriate.

2. Using understandable terminology is a teaching principle common to all age groups, not just older adults.

3. Obtaining a return demonstration is a teaching principle common to all age groups, not just older adults. This ensures that the learner has learned all the critical elements associated with the skill.

4. Reaction time will slow as one ages; therefore, older adults need more time

to process and respond to information or perform a skill. In addition, some older adults may have less energy, experience more fatigue, and may need shorter, frequent learning sessions.

6. 1. Learning is encouraged when positive behaviors are reinforced with a reward. However, food as a reward should be avoided in this scenario because it may foster old habits that contributed to the original weight gain. For people with an internal locus of control, rewards should center on recognition of personal achievement, such as pleasing oneself, returning to a usual lifestyle, avoiding complications, and, in this scenario, losing weight. For the person with an external locus of control, rewards might center on privileges or praise received from pleasing significant others or members of the health-care team.
2. Although exercise is an important component of any weight-loss program, exercise alone will not determine the success or failure of a weight-loss program.
3. This is a dependent function of the nurse and requires a primary health-care provider's order. In addition, an 800-calorie diet is too few calories to acquire basic nutrients to maintain adequate health. Weight-loss diets should be between 1200 and 1500 calories for women and between 1500 and 1800 calories for men.
4. Setting realistic goals is important to the success of a weight-loss program. Because achieving success is dependent largely on motivation, the teacher and patient should design goals that demonstrate immediate progress or growth. One strategy is to design numerous realistic short-term intermediary goals that are achieved more easily than one long-term goal.

7. 1. The nurse has been doing this and it has not been effective. A reassessment is necessary.
2. The patient already knows the technique of how to administer the injection. The issue is the patient is reluctant to self-administer the injection.
3. When a teaching plan is ineffective, the nurse must gather more data and revise the teaching plan to achieve the desired goal.
4. This promotes dependency and prevents the patient from becoming self-sufficient.

8. 1. The terms questionnaire and survey are used interchangeably to describe a type of evaluation tool designed to gather data about a topic. This method is used to obtain information, such as feedback regarding an educational program.
2. A post-test is not a questionnaire. A post-test is an examination given to assess cognitive learning after an educational program is completed.
3. A case study is not a questionnaire. A case study is a teaching tool that presents a scenario and a sequence of data to which the learner is required to analyze and respond.
4. A focus group is not a questionnaire. A focus group is designed to gather opinions and suggestions from a group of people about a particular topic using a discussion, not survey, format.

9. 1. The role-playing technique is unlikely to be used by adults preparing to retire. Role-playing is most often used when learning parenting and other interpersonal skills.
2. Men who are unwilling to admit that they have a drinking problem are not demonstrating readiness to learn. In addition, role-playing requires a person to assume a role for the purpose of learning a new behavior. These men are demonstrating an unwillingness to learn a new behavior.
3. A group of adolescents should benefit most from role-playing. Role-playing provides a safe environment in which to practice interpersonal skills. It enables individuals to rehearse what should be said, learn to respond to the emotional environment, and experience the pressures of the person playing the peer using drugs.
4. The role-playing technique is unlikely to be used by adults preparing for knee replacement surgery. Role-playing is most often used when learning parenting and other interpersonal skills.

10. 1. The fourth-grade reading level is too low for medical material. Research demonstrates that the average reading level is higher than fourth grade.

2. The eighth-grade reading level is too high a reading level for educational medical material. Randomized studies demonstrate that only 22% of individuals requiring health teaching are able to profit from written health materials on the eighth-grade reading level.
3. The 10th-grade reading level is too high a reading level for educational medical material. Twenty percent of Americans read at or below the fifth-grade reading level and are considered functionally illiterate.
4. **Randomized studies demonstrate that the average reading level of individuals who need health teaching is 6.8 grades of schooling.**

11. 1. **Learners progress through a program at their own pace viewing informational material, answering questions, and receiving immediate feedback. Some programs feature simulated situations that require critical thinking and a response. Correct responses are rationalized, praise is offered, and incorrect responses trigger an explanation of why the wrong answer is wrong and offer encouragement to try again. This is a superior teaching strategy for the learner who may find that group lessons are paced either too fast or too slowly for effective learning.**
2. Computer-assisted instruction (CAI) is not the least inexpensive teaching strategy. CAI requires a computer, keyboard, and station; software; technical support to install, maintain, and repair equipment; and a computer-literate teaching staff to preview, select, and implement CAI programs.
3. Although individual CAI programs often include pre- and post-testing components, this is not the greatest advantage of CAI as a teaching strategy.
4. Although CAI programs generally are well organized in a programmed instruction (step-by-step) format, this is not the greatest advantage of using CAI as a teaching strategy.

12. 1. Demonstrations generally are used for teaching a skill. Skills involve learning about equipment, rationales, and sequencing multiple steps and are too cognitively complex for the developmental abilities of a preschooler. A teaching method in another option is more age appropriate for a preschooler.
2. **Coloring books are the best approach because they require preschoolers to be active participants in their own learning. In addition, the child has a product to keep and be proud of, it reduces anxiety associated with learning because coloring is an activity most preschoolers are familiar with, and it is within a preschooler's cognitive level.**
3. Preschoolers are just beginning to interact with peers, have a short attention span, and get distracted easily, and therefore need a one-on-one relationship with the teacher. The teacher facilitates the learning specifically for the individual, keeps the learner focused, and provides reinforcement on the learner's cognitive level. Other age-specific strategies include games; storybooks; the use of dolls, puppets, or toys; and role-playing.
4. A video requires concentration and an attention span that may be beyond the developmental abilities of a preschooler.

13. 1. This scenario is not an example of a continuing education (CE) program. Continuing education refers to formal professional development experiences designed to enhance the knowledge or skills of the learner.
2. **Inservice programs generally are provided by health-care agencies to reinforce current knowledge and skills or provide new information about such issues as policies, theory, skills, practice, or equipment.**
3. This scenario is not an example of a certification program. The American Nurses Association has a certification program in which nurses can demonstrate minimum competence in specialty areas. Achievement of certification demonstrates advanced expertise and a commitment to ensuring competence.
4. This scenario is not an example of an orientation program. An orientation program is provided by a health-care agency to introduce new employees to the policies, procedures, departments, services, table of organization, expectations, equipment, and so on, within the agency.

14. 1. Assessing intelligence by a nurse is a subjective assessment that is difficult to perform. Declining functional abilities, debilitating diseases, pain, and stress may impair the intellectual functioning of some individuals.

2. Although it is important to assess a patient's experience before implementing a teaching plan, of the options offered it is not the first thing the nurse should do.
3. **If the patient does not recognize the need to learn or value the information to be learned, the patient will not be ready to learn.**
4. Although it is important to assess a patient's strengths before implementing a teaching plan, of the options offered, it is not the first thing the nurse should do.

15. 1. Although fear will affect the success of a teaching program and will need to be assessed and modifications employed, it is not the factor that will have the greatest impact on the future success of a teaching program. Fear initially causes change; however, as fear subsides a person often returns to the previous behavior.

2. **Of all the options presented, the patient in denial is the person least ready and motivated to learn. The patient in denial is unable to recognize the need for the learning.**
3. Fatigue is a physiological, not psychosocial, response to an illness. When teaching, the nurse must assess the patient's stamina and modify the teaching program so as not to unduly strain the patient and yet meet the objectives.
4. Although assessing for anxiety is important, it is not the factor that has the greatest impact on the future success of a teaching program. Mild anxiety is motivating. Moderate anxiety will motivate a patient to learn but may require the nurse to keep concepts and approaches simple. The person with moderate anxiety may need to be refocused and have distractions minimized to facilitate learning. If severe anxiety or panic is present, the teaching program will have to be postponed until the patient is less anxious.

16. 1. **The learner must recognize that the need exists and that the material to be learned is valuable. Motivation is the most important factor influencing learning.**

2. Although setting goals within the patient's value system is important, it is not the first thing the nurse should do before implementing a teaching plan.
3. Although the teacher should identify a patient's learning style, a variety of teaching methods, not just the patient's preference, should be used. This ensures that as many senses as possible are stimulated when learning, thereby increasing the probability of a successful outcome to the learning.
4. Although supportive individuals (e.g., family members and friends) can assist in helping the patient maintain a positive mental attitude and reinforce learning, another option has a higher priority.

17. 1. Teaching and learning involve one or all domains of learning (e.g., cognitive, affective, and psychomotor) and do not move from one to the other in progressive order.

2. Teaching methods that are formal or informal are equally effective. The key is to select the approach that is most likely to be effective for the individual learner. This depends on a variety of factors, such as intelligence, content to be taught, learning style preferences, available resources, reading level, and so on.
3. **When moving from the simple to the complex, a person works at integrating and incorporating the less complex, new learning into one's body of knowledge and understanding before moving on to more complex information. Complex material is best learned when easily understood aspects of the topic are presented first as a foundation for the more complex aspects.**
4. There is no documented principle that supports the need to present content in the direction of broad to specific rather than specific to broad. Each individual patient and the information to be taught will influence the direction in which content is taught.

18. 1. An explanation is not the best approach to teach a psychomotor skill. An explanation uses words to describe a behavior that the learner then has to attempt to perform.

2. **A demonstration is the best strategy for teaching a psychomotor skill. A demonstration is an actual performance of the skill by the teacher who is acting as a role model. A demonstration**

usually is followed by a return demonstration. The learner can imitate the teacher during a return demonstration, ask questions, and receive feedback from the instructor.

3. Although a video provides a realistic performance of the skill, it does not allow for questions or feedback.
4. A brochure with pictures is too static and one-dimensional for teaching a psychomotor skill.

19. 1. This option reflects learning in the cognitive domain. Cognitive learning involves the intellect and requires thinking.

2. This option reflects learning in the affective domain. Affective learning is concerned with feelings, emotions, values, beliefs, and attitudes about the colostomy.

3. Providing a demonstration on colostomy care is an example of a teaching strategy in the psychomotor domain. The psychomotor domain is related to mastering a skill and requires the use of physical and motor activity.
4. Showing a videotape demonstrating colostomy care is an example of a teaching strategy in the psychomotor domain. It reflects a beginning awareness of the objects needed and steps to be implemented in a skill.

20. 1. Role-playing is no more or less fun than many other active and creative learning strategies.

2. This is not the reason for using role-playing. Media equipment can be used with role-playing.

3. Learning activities that actively engage the learner have been shown to be more effective as well as more fun than methods that do not actively engage the learner. When learners are actively involved, they assume more responsibility for their own learning and develop more self-interest in learning the content.

4. Role-playing is designed to support rehearsing a desired behavior in a safe environment. Although it may involve an opportunity to play another person, which allows one to view a situation from another vantage point, it is not the most important reason why role-playing is effective.

21. 1. Although religious affiliation may be important to know, it is only one part of a patient's sociocultural makeup. Another option has a higher priority.

2. Although the level of support is important to know, it is only one part of a patient's sociocultural makeup. Another option has a higher priority.
3. Although national origin is important to know, it is only one part of a patient's sociocultural makeup. In addition, nurses have to be careful not to make generalizations and stereotype an individual because of national origin, because each person is an individual.

4. Individuals have their own beliefs associated with cultural health practices, faith, diet, illness, death and dying, and lifestyle, which all have a major impact on health beliefs. Not all members of a culture have the same beliefs.

22. 3. The first step of the options presented involves determining the patient's desire to learn. If the patient does not recognize that the learning is important, the patient will not be invested in the learning process.

1. The second step of the options presented is determining if the patient is ready to learn. The patient may be motivated to learn, but if the patient is in pain or fatigued, the patient may not be able to focus on the learning.

2. The third step of the options presented is to implement a teaching plan by engaging the patient in planned learning activities.

4. The fourth step of the options presented is related to the concept of repetition of essential concepts to facilitate retention of learned information. Practice of psychomotor skills along with feedback from the nurse strengthens the learning and encourages independence.

5. The fifth step of the options presented is the evaluation of the patient's performance in light of stated goals. When evaluating a psychomotor skill the nurse observes the patient's implementation of the skill to ensure that steps in the skill (e.g., collects necessary equipment, follows standards of asepsis and safety, and recognizes

5. Speaking slowly is an appropriate intervention for a patient who has a hearing, not a vision, impairment.

35. 1. Although an illustration appeals to visual learners, this is not the primary reason why the nurse educator decided to present this illustration to reinforce content presented in the lecture.
2. The concept of positive reinforcement is not associated with presenting an illustration to reinforce learning. Positive reinforcement is associated with using praise and encouragement to enhance motivation. Research by Ivan Pavlov and B. F. Skinner presented the theory of positive reinforcement.
3. An internal or external locus of control is associated with motivational theory and is unrelated to the rationale for using graphics to explain complex information.
4. Research demonstrates that when illustrations are used in conjunction with reading content, learners outperform students who just read the content. Illustrations attract attention, facilitate retention of information, and improve understanding of complex content by creating a context.

and responds to problems associated with the procedure) are implemented according to principles.

23. 1. Identifying the expected properties of urine reflects learning on the knowledge level, which is the first of six levels of complexity in the cognitive domain.
2. Explaining the importance of producing urine reflects learning on the comprehension level, which is the second of six levels of complexity in the cognitive domain.
3. Recognizing when something is contaminated reflects learning on the application level, which is the third level of six levels of complexity within the cognitive domain.
4. When a learner compares achieved outcomes with planned outcomes, the learner is evaluating the effectiveness of the learning. This activity is evaluation, which is the highest level of the cognitive domain. It requires the nurse to compare, contrast, and differentiate information.
5. This is the highest level of learning in the cognitive domain. Contrasting laboratory results of urine testing with the expected range reflects learning on the evaluation level, which is the sixth and highest level of learning in the cognitive domain.

24. **1.** The patient's pulse, respirations, and blood pressure are all slightly increased. These adaptations probably are being caused by the release of catecholamines resulting from the pain the patient is experiencing. Moderate to severe pain will interfere with learning. The patient will have difficulty concentrating on the task at hand. The nurse should postpone the teaching session, administer the prescribed pain medication, and reassess the patient in 30 minutes. The teaching session can be reinstituted after the pain is reduced.
2. Teaching at this time is an inappropriate intervention.
3. Notifying the primary health-care provider is unnecessary. The patient's adaptations are common responses to the patient's physical status.
4. Waiting will delay meeting the patient's physical needs.

25. **1.** Simple vocabulary with as few syllables as possible along with short simple sentences is less confusing for a patient with a comprehension deficit.
2. For people who have a cognitive deficit, participating in a learning program often makes them feel overwhelmed and threatened. The teacher should provide a structured environment in which variables are controlled to reduce anxiety and support comprehension. The nurse should minimize ambiguity, provide a familiar environment, teach at the same time each day, limit environmental distractions, and provide simple learning materials.
3. Clarifying unclear words stated by the patient helps the nurse understand what the patient is saying. Patient concerns and questions must be addressed by the nurse.
4. Speaking directly in front of the patient helps the patient with impaired hearing, not the patient who has a cognitive deficit.
5. The patient does not need a hearing evaluation. The patient's problem is a cognitive deficit, not a hearing loss.

26. **1.** Verifying the order should be done first because a diet requires a primary health-care provider's order; following a specific diet is a dependent function of the nurse.
5. Assessing motivation is one of the most important factors influencing learning. The learner must recognize that the need exists and that the need will be addressed through the learning.
2. Determining food preferences is part of nursing assessment. Food preferences can then be included in the teaching plan about the low-calorie diet.
3. Details of the diet can be taught after the order is verified, motivation is determined, and preferences are identified.
4. Evaluation is the final step of teaching. A meal plan designed by the patient requires not just an understanding of the information but an ability to apply the information.

27. **1.** The person with an external locus of control is motivated by rewards that center on privileges, incentives, or

praise received from pleasing significant others or members of the health-care team. Watching television is a privilege in this situation.

2. Self-motivated behavior indicates an internal, not external, locus of control. People with an internal locus of control are motivated by personal internal rewards such as achieving a personal goal, pleasing oneself, returning to a usual lifestyle, and avoiding complications.
3. **Pleasing others precipitates feedback that is often viewed as positive by the recipient. Positive verbal or nonverbal communication from another is an external reward.**
4. Understanding the expected outcome of therapy is associated with recognizing the goal one is working to achieve; it does not describe an external locus of control.
5. A self-actualized adult is motivated by an internal locus of control. According to Maslow, the self-actualized person is an individual who has a need to develop to one's maximum potential and personally realize one's qualities and abilities.

28. 1. Limiting the length of sessions is unnecessary. Hearing is the problem, not fatigue.
2. **Written materials augment verbal teaching. The patient can review the written materials during and after the teaching session.**
3. **Varieties of teaching methods facilitate learning because multiple senses are stimulated. When we see, hear, and touch, learning is more effective than when we see or hear alone. In addition, research demonstrates that we remember only 10% of what we read, 20% of what we hear, 30% of what we see, 50% of what we see and hear, and 80% of what we say and do.**
4. Some patients who are hearing impaired lip-read. Facing the patient enables the patient to see the nurse's lips clearly.
5. A group setting is the least desirable teaching format for hearing-impaired individuals. One-on-one learning sessions limit background noise and distractions that hinder learning. In addition, a one-on-one session allows for individual feedback that ensures that the message is received as intended.

29. 1. Accepting something indicates learning in the affective, not psychomotor, domain. Learning in the affective domain includes things such as feelings, emotions, and attitudes.
2. Explaining something indicates learning in the cognitive, not psychomotor, domain. Learning in the cognitive domain is reflected in the ability to understand the meaning of learned content.
3. **Performing an activity indicates learning in the psychomotor domain. Learning in the psychomotor domain is related to mastering a skill and requires motor activity.**
4. **Assembling something indicates learning in the psychomotor domain. Learning in the psychomotor domain is related to mastering a skill and requires motor activity.**
5. **Demonstrating something indicates learning in the psychomotor domain. Learning in the psychomotor domain is related to mastering a skill and requires motor activity.**

30. 1. This behavior is an example of learning in the cognitive, not affective, domain. Cognitive learning involves the intellect and requires thinking.
2. **Eating food on the ordered diet is an example of learning in the affective domain. When learning is incorporated into the learner's behavior because it is perceived as important, learning has occurred in the affective domain. Affective learning involves the expression of feelings and the changing of beliefs, attitudes, or values.**
3. Compiling a list of permitted foods is an example of learning in the cognitive, not affective, domain. Cognitive learning involves the intellect and requires thinking.
4. Asking questions is not an outcome demonstrating learning. This is an example of a question a learner might ask when learning content in the cognitive domain. Cognitive learning involves the intellect and requires thinking.
5. **Avoiding foods high in sugar is an example of learning in the affective domain. When learning is incorporated into the learner's behavior because it is perceived as important, learning has occurred in the affective domain. Affective learning involves the expression of feelings and the changing of beliefs, attitudes, or values.**

31. 1. Docusate sodium is a stool softener and is unrelated to the activity of bathing. Teaching the patient about skin assessment and skin care is best performed during a bath.
2. **An excellent time for the nurse to teach the patient about docusate sodium, a medication that promotes bowel elimination, is when the patient is being assisted to the toilet.**
3. Docusate sodium is a stool softener and is unrelated to the activity of monitoring a patient's daily weight. Daily weights are taken to assess fluid balance.
4. Docusate sodium is a stool softener and is unrelated to a dressing change of a pressure ulcer.
5. **During medication administration is a perfect time for the nurse to educate a patient about the medications that the patient is receiving.**

32. 3. **The first step in planning a teaching plan is to identify the information that the learner must acquire. This step is accomplished by formulating realistic, measurable learning goals.**
4. **The second step in planning a teaching plan is organizing the information in an appropriate sequence to be presented.**
1. **The third step in planning a teaching plan is the selection of the teaching strategies to be employed based on the advantages and disadvantages of each strategy and which is best to achieve the learning goals.**
5. **The fourth step in planning a teaching plan is to develop instructional materials that will reinforce and supplement information provided in the class.**
2. **The teacher should develop a method to evaluate whether learning goals are met. Post-tests, written exercises, questionnaires, surveys, and direct observation of performance are some examples of evaluation methods.**

33. 1. **Sensory impairment results from the aging process, which must be considered when planning a teaching plan for an older adult. Aging causes such changes as: a reduced ability to focus or accommodate because of reduced elasticity of the lens of the eye; a narrowing of the visual field; increased opacification of the lens that causes cataracts with accompanying blurring of vision and increased sensitivity to glare; a decrease in the ability to hear high-frequency sounds; and an increase in the keratin content of cerumen that causes an accumulation of cerumen in the middle ear and thus endangers hearing.**
2. **Various physiological changes of aging have an impact on the rate of learning (e.g., declines in sensory perception and speed of mental processing and more time needed for recall), requiring the use of multisensory teaching strategies and a repetitive approach. In addition, older adults may have less physical and emotional stamina because of more chronic illnesses, so they may require shorter and more frequent learning sessions.**
3. Although some older adults may experience a decline in short-term memory, they are not less intelligent. When older adults experience a decline in sensory function (e.g., vision, hearing), they may feel ashamed or frustrated, causing withdrawal. Behaviors reflective of withdrawal may be misperceived as a decline in intelligence.
4. This is not necessarily true. Individuals usually have learning preferences that persist throughout life.
5. Older adults generally are not resistant to change. Some older adults may be less motivated to learn if they believe that death is near. However, in this situation when older adults are shown how learning will improve their quality of life and independence, they are motivated to learn.

34. 1. **An automatic-stop syringe ensures that an appropriate dose of insulin can be prepared despite a patient's vision impairment.**
2. **Large print magnifies the written information to a size that may facilitate reading by the patient who is vision impaired.**
3. **Audio learning materials use the sense of hearing rather than sight to promote the teaching-learning process.**
4. Enunciating each word clearly is an appropriate intervention for a patient who has a hearing, not a vision, impairment.

and responds to problems associated with the procedure) are implemented according to principles.

23. 1. Identifying the expected properties of urine reflects learning on the knowledge level, which is the first of six levels of complexity in the cognitive domain.
2. Explaining the importance of producing urine reflects learning on the comprehension level, which is the second of six levels of complexity in the cognitive domain.
3. Recognizing when something is contaminated reflects learning on the application level, which is the third level of six levels of complexity within the cognitive domain.
4. When a learner compares achieved outcomes with planned outcomes, the learner is evaluating the effectiveness of the learning. This activity is evaluation, which is the highest level of the cognitive domain. It requires the nurse to compare, contrast, and differentiate information.
5. This is the highest level of learning in the cognitive domain. Contrasting laboratory results of urine testing with the expected range reflects learning on the evaluation level, which is the sixth and highest level of learning in the cognitive domain.

24. 1. The patient's pulse, respirations, and blood pressure are all slightly increased. These adaptations probably are being caused by the release of catecholamines resulting from the pain the patient is experiencing. Moderate to severe pain will interfere with learning. The patient will have difficulty concentrating on the task at hand. The nurse should postpone the teaching session, administer the prescribed pain medication, and reassess the patient in 30 minutes. The teaching session can be reinstituted after the pain is reduced.
2. Teaching at this time is an inappropriate intervention.
3. Notifying the primary health-care provider is unnecessary. The patient's adaptations are common responses to the patient's physical status.
4. Waiting will delay meeting the patient's physical needs.

25. 1. Simple vocabulary with as few syllables as possible along with short simple sentences is less confusing for a patient with a comprehension deficit.
2. For people who have a cognitive deficit, participating in a learning program often makes them feel overwhelmed and threatened. The teacher should provide a structured environment in which variables are controlled to reduce anxiety and support comprehension. The nurse should minimize ambiguity, provide a familiar environment, teach at the same time each day, limit environmental distractions, and provide simple learning materials.
3. Clarifying unclear words stated by the patient helps the nurse understand what the patient is saying. Patient concerns and questions must be addressed by the nurse.
4. Speaking directly in front of the patient helps the patient with impaired hearing, not the patient who has a cognitive deficit.
5. The patient does not need a hearing evaluation. The patient's problem is a cognitive deficit, not a hearing loss.

26. 1. Verifying the order should be done first because a diet requires a primary health-care provider's order; following a specific diet is a dependent function of the nurse.
5. Assessing motivation is one of the most important factors influencing learning. The learner must recognize that the need exists and that the need will be addressed through the learning.
2. Determining food preferences is part of nursing assessment. Food preferences can then be included in the teaching plan about the low-calorie diet.
3. Details of the diet can be taught after the order is verified, motivation is determined, and preferences are identified.
4. Evaluation is the final step of teaching. A meal plan designed by the patient requires not just an understanding of the information but an ability to apply the information.

27. 1. The person with an external locus of control is motivated by rewards that center on privileges, incentives, or

praise received from pleasing significant others or members of the health-care team. Watching television is a privilege in this situation.

2. Self-motivated behavior indicates an internal, not external, locus of control. People with an internal locus of control are motivated by personal internal rewards such as achieving a personal goal, pleasing oneself, returning to a usual lifestyle, and avoiding complications.
3. **Pleasing others precipitates feedback that is often viewed as positive by the recipient. Positive verbal or nonverbal communication from another is an external reward.**
4. Understanding the expected outcome of therapy is associated with recognizing the goal one is working to achieve; it does not describe an external locus of control.
5. A self-actualized adult is motivated by an internal locus of control. According to Maslow, the self-actualized person is an individual who has a need to develop to one's maximum potential and personally realize one's qualities and abilities.

28. 1. Limiting the length of sessions is unnecessary. Hearing is the problem, not fatigue.
2. **Written materials augment verbal teaching. The patient can review the written materials during and after the teaching session.**
3. **Varieties of teaching methods facilitate learning because multiple senses are stimulated. When we see, hear, and touch, learning is more effective than when we see or hear alone. In addition, research demonstrates that we remember only 10% of what we read, 20% of what we hear, 30% of what we see, 50% of what we see and hear, and 80% of what we say and do.**
4. Some patients who are hearing impaired lip-read. Facing the patient enables the patient to see the nurse's lips clearly.
5. A group setting is the least desirable teaching format for hearing-impaired individuals. One-on-one learning sessions limit background noise and distractions that hinder learning. In addition, a one-on-one session allows for individual feedback that ensures that the message is received as intended.

29. 1. Accepting something indicates learning in the affective, not psychomotor, domain. Learning in the affective domain includes things such as feelings, emotions, and attitudes.
2. Explaining something indicates learning in the cognitive, not psychomotor, domain. Learning in the cognitive domain is reflected in the ability to understand the meaning of learned content.
3. **Performing an activity indicates learning in the psychomotor domain. Learning in the psychomotor domain is related to mastering a skill and requires motor activity.**
4. **Assembling something indicates learning in the psychomotor domain. Learning in the psychomotor domain is related to mastering a skill and requires motor activity.**
5. **Demonstrating something indicates learning in the psychomotor domain. Learning in the psychomotor domain is related to mastering a skill and requires motor activity.**

30. 1. This behavior is an example of learning in the cognitive, not affective, domain. Cognitive learning involves the intellect and requires thinking.
2. **Eating food on the ordered diet is an example of learning in the affective domain. When learning is incorporated into the learner's behavior because it is perceived as important, learning has occurred in the affective domain. Affective learning involves the expression of feelings and the changing of beliefs, attitudes, or values.**
3. Compiling a list of permitted foods is an example of learning in the cognitive, not affective, domain. Cognitive learning involves the intellect and requires thinking.
4. Asking questions is not an outcome demonstrating learning. This is an example of a question a learner might ask when learning content in the cognitive domain. Cognitive learning involves the intellect and requires thinking.
5. **Avoiding foods high in sugar is an example of learning in the affective domain. When learning is incorporated into the learner's behavior because it is perceived as important, learning has occurred in the affective domain. Affective learning involves the**

expression of feelings and the changing of beliefs, attitudes, or values.

31. 1. Docusate sodium is a stool softener and is unrelated to the activity of bathing. Teaching the patient about skin assessment and skin care is best performed during a bath.

2. An excellent time for the nurse to teach the patient about docusate sodium, a medication that promotes bowel elimination, is when the patient is being assisted to the toilet.

3. Docusate sodium is a stool softener and is unrelated to the activity of monitoring a patient's daily weight. Daily weights are taken to assess fluid balance.

4. Docusate sodium is a stool softener and is unrelated to a dressing change of a pressure ulcer.

5. During medication administration is a perfect time for the nurse to educate a patient about the medications that the patient is receiving.

32. 3. The first step in planning a teaching plan is to identify the information that the learner must acquire. This step is accomplished by formulating realistic, measurable learning goals.

4. The second step in planning a teaching plan is organizing the information in an appropriate sequence to be presented.

1. The third step in planning a teaching plan is the selection of the teaching strategies to be employed based on the advantages and disadvantages of each strategy and which is best to achieve the learning goals.

5. The fourth step in planning a teaching plan is to develop instructional materials that will reinforce and supplement information provided in the class.

2. The teacher should develop a method to evaluate whether learning goals are met. Post-tests, written exercises, questionnaires, surveys, and direct observation of performance are some examples of evaluation methods.

33. 1. Sensory impairment results from the aging process, which must be considered when planning a teaching plan for an older adult. Aging causes such changes as: a reduced ability to focus or accommodate because of reduced elasticity of the lens of the eye; a narrowing of the visual field; increased opacification of the lens that causes cataracts with accompanying blurring of vision and increased sensitivity to glare; a decrease in the ability to hear high-frequency sounds; and an increase in the keratin content of cerumen that causes an accumulation of cerumen in the middle ear and thus endangers hearing.

2. Various physiological changes of aging have an impact on the rate of learning (e.g., declines in sensory perception and speed of mental processing and more time needed for recall), requiring the use of multisensory teaching strategies and a repetitive approach. In addition, older adults may have less physical and emotional stamina because of more chronic illnesses, so they may require shorter and more frequent learning sessions.

3. Although some older adults may experience a decline in short-term memory, they are not less intelligent. When older adults experience a decline in sensory function (e.g., vision, hearing), they may feel ashamed or frustrated, causing withdrawal. Behaviors reflective of withdrawal may be misperceived as a decline in intelligence.

4. This is not necessarily true. Individuals usually have learning preferences that persist throughout life.

5. Older adults generally are not resistant to change. Some older adults may be less motivated to learn if they believe that death is near. However, in this situation when older adults are shown how learning will improve their quality of life and independence, they are motivated to learn.

34. 1. An automatic-stop syringe ensures that an appropriate dose of insulin can be prepared despite a patient's vision impairment.

2. Large print magnifies the written information to a size that may facilitate reading by the patient who is vision impaired.

3. Audio learning materials use the sense of hearing rather than sight to promote the teaching-learning process.

4. Enunciating each word clearly is an appropriate intervention for a patient who has a hearing, not a vision, impairment.

5. Speaking slowly is an appropriate intervention for a patient who has a hearing, not a vision, impairment.

35. 1. Although an illustration appeals to visual learners, this is not the primary reason why the nurse educator decided to present this illustration to reinforce content presented in the lecture.
2. The concept of positive reinforcement is not associated with presenting an illustration to reinforce learning. Positive reinforcement is associated with using praise and encouragement to enhance motivation. Research by Ivan Pavlov and B. F. Skinner presented the theory of positive reinforcement.
3. An internal or external locus of control is associated with motivational theory and is unrelated to the rationale for using graphics to explain complex information.
4. Research demonstrates that when illustrations are used in conjunction with reading content, learners outperform students who just read the content. Illustrations attract attention, facilitate retention of information, and improve understanding of complex content by creating a context.